Now That You've Had Your Baby

How to Feel Better and Happier Than Ever After Childbirth

GIDEON G. PANTER, M.D.

and

SHIRLEY MOTTER LINDE, M.S.

David McKay Company, Inc.
New York

To W. P. H.

Library of Congress Cataloging in Publication Data

Panter, Gideon G.
  Now that you've had your baby.

  Includes index.
  1. Puerperium. 2. Puerperium—Psychological
aspects. 3. Infants (Newborn)—Care and hygiene.
I. Linde, Shirley Motter, joint author.
II. Title.
RG801.P36   618.6'02'40431   75–29302
ISBN 0–679–50497–4

1894347

CONTENTS

A Message from the Authors

The purpose of this book is to show you how to get yourself
back together again—physically and emotionally—after
childbirth, and to help you and your husband start out as
relaxed parents.

There are books and courses on pregnancy and childbirth.
And books on child care, infant nutrition, and the psychol-
ogy of infants and children.

But there are no courses about what happens to the parents immediately after childbirth, no classes to tell the new
mother and father how to meet their *new feelings and responsibilities* when they get home from the hospital, no guide to
prepare new parents for the dramatic changes in their lives
that occur with a brand-new baby.

And especially, there are no books that cover the special
needs of women after birth, for both the period in the hospital and the months thereafter. It is during this time of transition, of emotional and physical change, of frustration, and of

new duties that women have the most feelings of inadequacy. And yet it is the period when they have the least support and help.

The new mother's awesome feeling of total responsibility is usually overwhelming, and some of the reactions and emotions within the woman can be confusing and even frightening to her and to the new father.

And while the new mother is attempting to cope with these feelings, her body and metabolism are changing dramatically. The husband, too, and the baby are changing from day to day.

Over and over, patients who have just given birth have asked for information to help them. This book is designed to provide that help, to give the mother and father practical, down-to-earth advice, and to do it in language the ordinary reader can easily understand.

No one can sit down and really tell someone else all at once what coming home with a new baby is about. As each day comes, a new mother needs detailed explanations and advice to which she can refer over and over again as the need arises. As a new mother, you will find that certain situations during the postpartum period are gracefully met and enjoyed, while other events that apparently were no problem to other mothers will be perplexing and troublesome to you.

In this book we have attempted to tell you the story of what is happening to you the few first weeks and months after delivery and after coming home with a new baby. We discuss the continuum of changes and how to deal with them. We have dealt with particulars in order to give you a greater awareness of your feelings and of the changes that take place, not in the baby, but in you. The book is designed to be a source to which you can refer for specific answers and for detailed explanations, as well as for general concepts, to make the transition period smoother and more efficient.

You can read it in preparation for this special time in your life, and it will be a manual to which you and your husband can refer continually as you develop in the transition from birth to relaxed parenthood.

The questions dealt with are those obtained from thousands of women who have asked these actual questions of their doctors during this troublesome period. The responses are straightforward doctor-to-patient answers, plus added narratives and case histories.

In most cases throughout the book we have referred to the baby as "it" simply in order to avoid using "he" or the cumbersome "he-she" "him-her" pronoun forms, although we would not expect you to refer to the baby in this manner.

So this is not a baby book about how to make formula and how to change diapers. This is a guide to becoming physically and emotionally trim again, a guide through the shaky, gingerly taken first steps of what we hope will become relaxed motherhood.

Gideon Panter
Shirley Linde

NOW THAT
YOU'VE HAD
YOUR BABY

1

Welcome to Motherhood . . . What Do I Do Now?

"Suddenly you're somebody's mother! You look at this tiny, wrinkled, helpless thing and realize *you* are its mother . . ."

It was a new mother talking in a group session. They were all new mothers meeting to talk over their problems.

"My doctor just didn't prepare me! He didn't tell me what to *really* expect, how I would feel. I had no ideas of what the major problems would be with the baby or with myself." . . . Karen H., mother of three months.

"The doctor told me about vitamins and when the baby's umbilical cord would fall off. And said no sex. But he didn't tell me about the crying, about the responsibility, about the feeling alone, about the insecurity of being a new mother. He said to call him with any problems. But I didn't. I figured he was too busy. I felt completely isolated and on my own." . . . It was Sandra, mother of Bobby.

"Everything had been building to this fantastic thing—motherhood. How I was going to come home with this baby and it was going to be tremendous and I was going to feel so changed and so different. And I didn't. I didn't feel different one bit. In fact, I couldn't even relate to the baby. It was a very pretty little thing, but I didn't have any tremendous feelings for it. *I* needed to be taken care of. Me! I was very frightened, and nobody had prepared me for those feelings!" . . . It was Sally. Now a happy mother. Before, she had been very scared.

"I remember in the hospital they brought me the baby and I said, 'Wait a minute, what do I do now?' And then when I came home I suddenly realized the hand that rocked the cradle was my own. If only I had had somebody to talk to!" . . . Mildred.

These new mothers talking were a few of the hundreds we listened to in writing this book.

Mildred was nearly in tears. She admitted she had been insecure, lonely, and afraid. And she was angry at herself and feeling *guilty* because she was insecure, lonely, and afraid.

What she hadn't known was that she was not alone. She didn't know that instant motherhood doesn't just happen—to anyone. That nearly every woman goes through real problems during the first few weeks and months of being a new mother.

Important changes happen to a baby as it goes from the soft, shielding home in the uterus to the noisy, bright, outside world. It is thrust, buffeted, shoved, and squeezed under tremendous pressure through the birth canal into the world. Major blood vessels close off since it no longer gets oxygen and food from its mother. Other blood vessels open to connect its own lungs to its heart. Its lungs expand with the first breath of air. It sees its first light, hears its first sound, feels things against its skin for the first time. Its digestion starts to function on its own.

Big changes.

But the mother experiences just as many changes—enormous changes—just not so evident. She has physical changes, hormone changes, mental changes, a new life-style thrust upon her, with responsibilities she never knew before.

Nine months of physical changes to the new mother's body and to its organs are being undone in just a few weeks as her body returns to normal. And simultaneously, she must learn to cope with her baby, with herself, with her new relationships to her family and to her husband, and to the new impact she makes upon the world in her new role.

This book will be about the new mother and the changes in *her* life from birth through her passage beyond the first trying months.

The postpartum period is as important to motherhood as the pregnancy itself, and is almost as miraculous.

Postpartum means *after delivery.* Doctors call it *puerperium.* It starts the minute labor ends. And at no other time in her entire life do a woman's tissues and emotions change so much in such a short time.

And new mothers usually have very little help with their changes.

The obstetrician is busy. Or the new mother doesn't even know what to ask him. The nurses are busy. The husband is as insecure and innocent about what is happening as the new mother.

Today the obstetrician discharges his patient on the third or fourth day, perhaps even earlier. At that time he might sit down for five minutes at the bedside and tell the patient not to have sex and not to use tampons and not to take baths. He will say a few words about when she can leave the house and perhaps about driving a car, and he may review the essentials of breast-feeding. And then he will shake the patient's hand and tell her to call if she has any problems. Of course, she's not quite sure what *are* problems.

When women in the postpartum period were interviewed by a research team at Tulane University recently, it was found that the women had fairly adequate knowledge about the care of their infants, but knew little about the care of themselves.

Physicians must be aware of the mothers' physical and

emotional needs as well as the needs of the infants.

Feminist Betty Friedan once interviewed Julie Harris about having her baby. "It scared me," the actress said. "How could I take responsibility for someone else's life? What kind of mother would I be?"

That fear has been expressed by nearly every new mother to whom we talked.

The new mother has no one to turn to, no one to answer her questions.

Our experiences—as a doctor and as a woman searching for a doctor—have shown us the real needs of the new mother—needs that are not being met.

No matter how warm and friendly and great your doctor is, he is still a very busy man, he has many other patients, he doesn't know what you know and don't know, and he assumes you know many things you don't. And even if he wants to, he simply can't go over every single thing that might bother every new mother. And most important, he isn't *there*, right with you when you really need him, when you are discouraged or when you simply have a question.

How great it would be if you could have your doctor with you during this time, as somebody to turn to with questions, as a best friend and confidante, someone sympathetic who knows the momentary loneliness and frightening feelings you may have now. It would be grand to have someone who could answer questions you might have about how to get a flat stomach back again fast, how to breast-feed successfully, what to do about being tired, what you should eat or not eat, how long there will be bleeding, and when you can start to have sex again.

We've tried to design this book to answer all these questions, to be that medical friend. It not only has the information you need to know to truly get you back together again —better than ever before—but it's *on your side*. And it will help your husband too.

We know that with all the joys and happiness of having a baby, some of the adjustment can be difficult. And when you don't have 100-percent joy and happiness and instant mother instinct, you may feel guilty. Or you may become frightened at the sudden overwhelming responsibility, or wonder if you have the ability to share that responsibility as husband and wife.

You may want to work and not know what the effect on your baby will be, or how to handle it. You may have bad feelings toward the baby and feel guilty about them.

You may have found that when you were pregnant, you were the center of attention, you were treated tenderly, given a seat on the subway, smiled at sweetly, and catered to. Then suddenly you are removed from the center of the stage to the sidelines of diaper-washing and baby-burping.

You may have had a romantic vision of walking into the sunset in the joy of new motherhood, your baby and your husband at your side. Then came the reality. Pregnancy simply doesn't prepare you for the reality of coming home a new mother.

This book will try to fill the gap, will try to help you determine what is myth and reality, and will try to give you the kind of dialogue you would have with an understanding obstetrician if you had her or him with you all the time. It will give you the advice you should be getting from doctors, but almost never do.

Becoming a new mother now is different from what it used to be. Having the baby is about the same. But the transition period to relaxed motherhood—that's what is different.

Years ago, the new mother was kept in bed, usually in the hospital, for two or three weeks after the birth. Meals were brought to her and she was pampered by nurses or by her family. During that time she would be given instructions by the hospital nurses on how to sterilize formulas and on how to diaper and feed and clothe the baby. She only gradually learned of her baby's needs and personality and only slowly became active in her new role as mother.

Years ago, when the new mother came home, she found a milieu of helpers—either servants or relatives, including parents and parents-in-law, sisters and sisters-in-law. They helped to do chores and taught her how to care for the baby and they reassured her emotionally as she coped with new feelings and new insecurities. Or she might have had a baby nurse who knew just what to do.

The circumstances are totally different now. The "Scientific Approach" has been applied to the new mother. It has been found that early ambulation leads to less infection and fewer of the complications that result from prolonged bed rest. Mothers are led to the bathroom as soon as they return to their rooms after birth.

Hospital stays are shorter. Because of the increasing costs of medical care, hundreds of dollars are saved by shortening the hospital stay. But the trend to shorter hospitalization also came about because of an increasing psychological awareness —a concern for the patient who misses her home and perhaps other children, and a regard for the husband who wants to be with his family. Now it is not unusual for the new mother to be discharged on the third or fourth postpartum day.

When the new mother comes home, she is on her own. Her own mother may live and work in a far city, unable to leave to train her daughter in the specifics and vagaries of new motherhood. And her sister may be off in another city too. Today, the woman with a new baby is on her own.

We think today's new mothers are getting short shrift. We've brought together the facts to help them.

2

The Hospital

Labor and delivery are over. You lie in your hospital bed exhausted, groggy, but very very happy.

You are a mother. A mother!! The thought both terrifies and exhilarates you.

The greatest event in life is birth, and you have just been part of it.

It's a strange sensation now of being empty after feeling so filled and heavy for so long. You think about not just being an independent person from now on, but always having another soul depending on you for its help.

You look around the room—a different one from the one you were in when in labor, which now seems so long ago. You're in the same hospital gown, there are the same stiff, white sheets, the nightstand with the call button for the nurse next to you. But the room is bigger and cheerier. You notice your suitcase and clothes have been transferred and are hanging in the closet.

The nurse comes in, checks your pulse, takes your temperature, measures your blood pressure, and feels around your lower abdomen.

Later your obstetrician pops in beaming. "A beautiful baby! How do you feel?" He talks to you for a while, kneads your stomach some more, tells you to rest and catch some sleep, and is off.

You try to, and groggily you wonder about what has just happened and what the next few days will bring.

A time of thinking.

Somehow, as you lie in your hospital bed later and marvel over the enormity and significance of bringing another life into the world, many serious thoughts come to your mind. You probe the meaning of childbirth as a culmination of many of your dreams from girlhood on. What a marvelous, warm, welcome human being your child is.

And you think about this huge change in your life and what it will mean. How have you changed, or have you really changed at all?

What will be expected of you now by others? And by yourself? Will you be able to measure up?

You enter the period of new motherhood lying there thinking you aren't going to march with such sureness after all, despite all the classes you took, but will enter motherhood much more cautiously than you thought . . . with an uncertain and perhaps uneasy tread.

It is a time of introspection, of taking inventory, of soul-searching.

Your head begins to fill with memories and dreams and thinking through.

You relive your labor and delivery all over again, minute by minute, from the moment you felt the first pain, through the trip to the hospital. You remember the contractions, your husband holding your hand. You remember the ride down the corridor to the delivery room and the really big pushes, the convulsive contractions, that shook your whole body. And you remember seeing your new child for the first time.

And as your baby began its journey down through the

birth canal to a new world, so you too now are beginning a new journey to a new world as a parent.

But soon your thoughts rivet back to your baby again.

What happens to my baby after delivery?

The first order of business is to clear the baby's airway so that he can breathe and cry with no obstruction. Even as his head emerges from your vagina, the obstetrician or his assistant suctions out the baby's nose and mouth with a rubber suction bulb.

Sometimes the baby begins to cry on its own at this time in response to the rude shock it feels as it leaves your warm body and meets the cold air.

The new baby is then taken to a special crib called a resuscitator, where it is placed with its head tilted down. More suctioning of the air passages is done here. When the air passages are free, the baby is stimulated to cry if it is not crying already. Sometimes oxygen is given to the baby to help to revive it. And it is not slapped on its seat if a stimulus is needed; the obstetrician will strike a glancing blow on the soles of the baby's feet. Babies must hate that because it always starts their crying.

The umbilical cord is clamped closer to the baby and cut, and the baby is turned over to the nurse, who usually gives the parents a good look at this time.

What does the nurse do to my baby?

The nurse puts medicine in the baby's eyes in order to prevent any of the vaginal germs that are present from causing infection. This is primarily prevention against gonorrheal conjunctivitis, an eye infection that can cause blindness. It is not necessary if you have had cesarean section since the eyes of babies delivered that way are not exposed to vaginal organisms.

Next the baby receives an injection of vitamin K to help the clotting system of the blood develop. You can tell when that is done because babies react to that injection as they do to being slapped on their feet. It's a reassuring reaction.

The baby is then wrapped in a blanket and only a hard-hearted nurse would refuse to give you the baby to hold at that time.

What happens to me after the baby is born?

After your obstetrician turns the baby over to the delivery room team for the baby care we have discussed, he turns back to you and proceeds to help the placenta deliver itself. The placenta, or afterbirth, is that specialized organ that during pregnancy transferred nutrients and oxygen from you to the baby and waste products from the baby to you. The moment the baby is born, the placenta loses its usefulness.

The uterus usually contracts forcefully after the baby is born, and the placenta is expelled. The process is speeded and thus blood loss is reduced by giving the mother an injection to cause these contractions as the baby is born. You will feel the placenta emerging from the birth canal as a mild version of childbirth.

The stitches are then placed to close the episiotomy (the small incision made to ease the birth). If you are awake (and we hope that you are), you will usually be too excited to notice. But if you do, ask for more local anesthesia, just as you would tell the dentist when a tooth he is drilling begins to hurt.

The obstetrician will then congratulate you and your husband, who often is in the delivery room with you.

Why am I kept on the delivery floor after the delivery is completed?

It is very important that you be observed closely during the hour or two following delivery. This is a time when sudden swings in blood pressure can occur. This is the time when your anesthesia wears off, whether it be local or regional or general.

Your blood pressure, pulse, and temperature will be measured to be sure that you are normal. Your abdomen will be felt and squeezed gently to ascertain that your uterus is contracting well. If it does not, excessive blood loss can occur.

When it has been established that you are stable and recovering normally, you are sent to your room. Most hospitals will allow your husband to stay with you during this period of observation.

How do the doctors know my baby is normal?

Even before the umbilical cord is cut, the doctors in the delivery room are starting to examine your baby. They look at the skin color and take the pulse and temperature. They look over the entire body to see that muscles, bones, and face are normal.

How do I know my baby is normal?

Within the first minute of life your baby gets its first report card. Doctors check him or her in five major categories: heart rate, breathing, muscle tone, reflexes, and color. In each of these categories, the baby is graded from zero to two, and the total is added up. The total is called the Apgar score, named after the internationally known pediatrician Dr. Virginia Apgar.

"Is my baby all right?" Ninety-eight percent of the time, the answer is a resounding "Yes."

What can I expect in hospital routine?

The complications following delivery are rare, but when they occur they usually occur within a few days. These complications are postpartum hemorrhage, infections of the uterus and urinary systems, and sometimes elevated blood pressures.

For this reason you will be compulsively observed. Your temperature will be taken frequently, since it is often the first sign of infection. Your blood pressure and pulse will be measured, your sanitary pads looked at, which you will now be wearing for several weeks, and your abdomen kneaded.

Why is everybody always kneading my abdomen?

Your uterus is supposed to involute (get back to normal) at a given rate: every day it gets smaller. If it stops involuting, or begins to dilate or enlarge, excessive bleeding can occur.

When your tummy is kneaded, the uterus is being measured. And it is being massaged, which encourages it to contract more.

You can do this yourself, quite safely, and very effectively. Reach down and feel your uterus as a hard lump, just below your umbilicus (navel). Now massage, just as if you were feeling a grapefruit or lettuce to be sure it's not spoiled.

The aftereffects of anesthesia and what to do about them.

You will be kept on the delivery floor until the anesthesia has worn off. If you have had general anesthesia, you will probably also need a good nap to clear up your head and get a steady walk.

As local and regional anesthesias wear off, you might notice too sharp a transition from no pain to pain. Ask for a pain pill or shot if you wish help to get through the painful time.

How soon can I get out of bed?

There is no special rule here. It depends on how you feel after the delivery. This is often related to the length of your labor and how tired you might be, or to the type of anesthesia and to whether or not it has worn off.

Most mothers are ready to get out of bed by the time they have to urinate for the first time after the birth. But you must have assistance for your first venture. Ring for the nurse, no matter how well you feel, and ask her to walk you to the bathroom.

Your body has worked hard, and it is not unusual to feel unsteady. You may feel faint. Fortunately, any fainting that occurs at this time is usually a graceful, gentle swoon from which you recover immediately.

A typical day in the maternity ward.

You'll be a lot busier than you think. First of all, all those stories about how early you get up are basically true. You can count on being awakened at about seven thirty in the morning to have your temperature measured. You wash up, and the babies are soon brought in for nursing. Breakfast for you arrives anywhere between eight and eight thirty.

Then you will probably read the newspaper and you may

have a heat lamp treatment in the incision area where the stitches were made. An aide will change your bed linen and give you fresh water. An attendant will sweep the floor, empty trash, and straighten up. The nurse will come by to take your pulse and temperature and give you any prescribed medications. A vendor may go through with papers and magazines. Flowers may arrive. An aide comes in with juice. An intern or resident may stop by. You steal a nap.

The babies come back for their late morning feeding. Then another nap for you, followed by lunch. Then generally time for another nap. Now it's time for visitors. Babies again. Juice again. Perhaps a walk to the nursery window. Somewhere in between you work in more exercises, another heat lamp treatment, make out your birth announcements, take a shower, and comb your hair. Dinner tray. Babies again. Nurses again. Visitors again. Juice again. Babies again. And you fall asleep exhausted.

Can I have any fun in the hospital?

You certainly can. In fact, it's mostly fun. It is a time to get used to the baby, a time to meet other new mothers, a time to reflect on your feelings, a time to discuss feelings with the nurses and your husband and your doctor, and a time to learn the elements of baby care.

Talk to your nurses while you are in the hospital. They are there to answer your questions and to show you tricks in baby care and to teach you anything about your own body you want to know.

Things not to worry about that are perfectly natural in your new baby.

- Red, wrinkled skin. They all look like that. Like wrinkled, emaciated, ancient old men and women.
- White, cheesy-looking material on the skin. It's called vernix. It's left over from the coating that covered your baby's entire body for protection. It will wear off with a few washings.
- Molded head. Often in delivery the head is strangely shaped to fit through the birth canal. It will soon become rounded.

- Sneezing. It's common, clears the upper respiratory tract.
- Eyes out of focus, even crossed. He will focus in soon. In the meantime, the baby can see shapes and lights, and its eyes will follow a bright object or will squint or frown at a bright light.
- A violent, startled reaction to sound. Loud noises typically cause this reaction, often with arms and legs flailing wildly. The reaction is called the Moro reflex.
- Irregular breathing. Sometimes babies pant, sometimes gasp or hold their breath or breathe in long, slow breaths.
- Its eyes are blue, and your husband and you both have brown eyes. All babies have blue eyes at birth. Later they will develop their permanent color.
- Pulse beating in the head. All babies have soft spots in their skulls where the bones will not grow together for several months. You can often see the pulse of an artery in these areas.
- The baby is like a hairy ape. The fine hair that covers his ears, back, and shoulders is called lanugo. It will disappear shortly.
- Bowlegs. His legs may be bowed, or his feet may turn in different directions. They'll straighten.
- Bruises. If the face is puffy and bruised, it is showing the effects of a tight passage through the birth canal. Healing will be quick.
- Strawberry marks or blue spots. Strawberry marks, red and raised, usually disappear, though occasionally some last until school age. Port-wine stains, which are purple and flat, remain for life unless treated by plastic surgery or tattooing. Black children often have blue spots on the lower back or seat, which usually become smaller or completely disappear early in life.
- Swollen genitals and breasts. Hormones in the mother often affect the newborn infant. In fact, sometimes both boy and girl babies will secrete some milk, known as "witches' milk." Some newborn girls will even show a slight menstrual flow for a few days after birth.

Should I take milk of magnesia or cathartics offered in the hospital?

Some women have difficulty with constipation in the hospital or at home after delivery, so that many obstetric wards of hospitals offer some laxative routinely.

However, bowel movements are still among the most over-rated experiences in the hospital. They usually will happen with no special fanfare if you just forget about it.

Certainly milk of magnesia is safe. But if you are sure to have adequate fluid intake of at least three quarts (twelve glasses) of fluid every day in the hospital, you probably will have no problem. Your first bowel movement usually occurs about day four or five, which means there is no special reason for having it prior to your discharge from the hospital.

Other medications you may be given and what they are for.

Ergonovine is a medication to cause the uterus to contract. It hastens involution, and studies have shown that, in general, mothers who receive this drug after childbirth bleed less and have a lower risk of having a postpartum hemorrhage.

Ergonovine, often called by its trade name ergotrate, is a small, white pill given four times a day for about two days after delivery. When it causes contractions of the uterus, you feel them as cramps. It is completely safe for nursing mothers and is an insurance against hemorrhaging.

Pain medicines. Because of contractions after birth, which are often felt as painful cramps, and because the episiotomy will often hurt for a day or two, your doctor will prescribe something for pain. There are various forms of pain medicines that he can prescribe, and he will have ordered something safe for nursing mothers and appropriate to the pain he expects.

You usually have to ask for pain medicine, however. It is not given to you automatically. You should not hesitate to ask for it because it is safe and will enable you to rest better and thus regain your strength more rapidly.

Iron and vitamins. It is natural to bleed during and following a normal delivery. However, the bleeding removes iron from your body, and your iron stores were already reduced by the iron going into the baby, so it is important to take iron and vitamins after delivery. Often they are combined into one pill or capsule.

The capsules will also help to improve the vitamin and mineral content of the milk of nursing mothers.

Sleeping pills. Having a baby is an enormously invigorating experience and causes everyone involved to get high. Frequently the new mother is so stimulated by the experience that she is unable to sleep for the first night or two. Even if you have no difficulty in sleeping, ask for your sleeping pill for the first few nights, because your days will be filled with learning and adjustments that are best met if you are rested.

The sleeping pill ordered by your doctor is also safe for nursing mothers.

The perineum and episiotomy.

Even though you probably had an episiotomy, the birth of the baby caused a great deal of stretch of the vagina and also the muscles of the perineum (the "blank" area between your anus and vagina). In addition, there might be swelling of the vagina and vulva related to the forces and pressures during labor. You may notice this swelling between your legs during the first day or two when you are walking. This swelling will gradually subside. Muscles regain their tone as the stitches heal. Also, the cut edges of the episiotomy will be sensitive for a few days until healing has started.

It is very helpful to put an ice bag against the perineum whenever you are in bed during the first twenty-four hours after birth. This will help the swelling subside, much as an ice bag will on a bumped head or black eye. If the ice bag is not offered by the nurse on the postpartum floor, do not hesitate to ask for it.

It is also helpful to rinse your perineum with cool water after urinating or having a bowel movement. The urine residue on your perineum is often irritating.

After the first twenty-four hours, warm showers will feel wonderful as they soothe your bottom and help the muscles to relax. Much of the postpartum pain is due to a reflex tightening of your perineal muscles, which you tighten as a protective measure. These muscles are tightened so much that they can become spastic, much like a "charley horse." And warmth helps them to relax.

The perineal exercises we describe in the chapter on exercises help you to regain control of these muscles so that you can relax them as well as tighten them.

Heating lamp.

A simple heating lamp will probably be supplied by the hospital, or it can be nothing more than your bedside reading lamp put to good use. When shined on your perineum it will provide heat to stimulate blood flow and help healing of stitches, and to help spastic, tense muscles to relax.

And when shined on your nipples it will help to dry them and will speed healing of any cracking or sore spots.

When will the stitches come out?

Most obstetricians use stitch material that dissolves. This is called "cat gut," although it is manufactured chemically and has nothing to do with cats. The "gut" usually automatically dissolves at seven to ten days, so stitches do not have to be taken out by hand.

How soon can I take a shower?

You can take a shower as soon as you feel steady enough. And this also holds true after cesarean section. There is no need to keep the stitches dry; early showering does not increase the incidence of infection.

If you had a cesarean.

The main difference is that your intestines will be sluggish for a few days. The doctor and nurses will ask you if you have passed flatus (gas), since that is the signal that your intestines have become active again. When the flatus passes, your diet will be advanced, and intravenous fluids routinely given cesarean patients will usually be discontinued.

What you need to know about being Rh negative.

About 15 percent of women have Rh negative blood. This means that they are lacking a coating on their blood cells called the Rh factor.

If a woman who is Rh negative gives birth to a baby who is Rh positive, or even miscarries or aborts an Rh positive fetus, she can develop an allergy to Rh positive blood. If this allergy is allowed to develop, it will act on her next Rh positive baby and can cause serious damage.

Fortunately, there is a special vaccine available now that prevents the allergy from developing. Whenever an Rh negative mother has an abortion or gives birth to an Rh positive baby, she gets an injection of this vaccine to keep the allergy from developing, thus protecting the next child.

This vaccine is called Rho Gam and it will be given to you in the hospital if you are Rh negative and your baby is Rh positive.

The birth certificate and what you need to know.

Don't be nervous about the birth certificate. Someone will give you a form on which you are to fill in the baby's name. Don't worry if you haven't decided or if you decide that you wish to change it at a later date because Aunt Mary thinks the name is too masculine or too feminine, or because the name is too common. (Michelle and Jennifer were the most common girls' names of 1973; everyone seemed to be named Ryan in 1974.)

For a small filing fee, usually one or two dollars, you can change the birth certificate whenever you wish.

To circumcise or not to circumcise.

Years ago people did not have ready access to baths or showers. Babies who were not circumcised tended to have frequent infections due to accumulated debris under the foreskin. But now everyone has access to bathing.

Doctors have been arguing for years whether it is best medically to circumcise or not to circumcise. The baby should probably match his father and this should be your

main rationale for choosing circumcision. Little boys frequently see their fathers urinating. Toilet training is frequently accomplished by following this example. They want
to grow up to be like their fathers, and the sense of identification is helped if they match.

How to handle visitors.

Visitors to the maternity floor are usually limited. Frequently there is special time for husbands only.

If the hospital does allow other visitors, have them if you
wish, but also feel free to say you really would enjoy them
more if they waited until you were home in a few days.

No visitor should be welcome unless he telephones first to
find out the best time to see you.

No visitors should stay longer than you want, and you
should not hesitate to say so if you feel it is time to rest.
Never have more than a couple of visitors at a time. It is
simply too tiring. If you're basically shy or don't like to hurt
people's feelings, simply apologize and say your doctor is
very firm, and you're very sorry but he simply won't allow
you to see visitors until you go home.

No visitors should ever be thoughtless or stupid enough to
show up with a cold. If they do, get them out fast.

What you should have at the hospital.

Chances are you had your suitcase packed carefully for
days—maybe weeks—before you went to the hospital. But if
not, here is a checklist so you can have your husband bring
in whatever you don't have.

Something to sleep in if you hate hospital gowns. The one
advantage to the hospital gown is that the hospital launders
it. But if you really hate them, bring your own nightgowns
or pajamas. Something with buttons down the front makes
nursing easier.

A bed jacket. If you decide to put up with hospital gowns,
a top of your own is some improvement. Hospital rooms are
usually so warm, though, that you will probably end up not
wearing it. Frankly, unless you already own one, we suggest
you don't bother.

A robe and slippers. A must, because you will want to walk around the halls both to see the baby in the nursery and to get some exercise and work off any restlessness. Socks if your feet tend to get cold.

A nursing bra. Makes nursing much easier. Buy a good one with proper support, with plastic inserts for protection from moisture, or put gauze pads in the cups to absorb the milk that sometimes leaks from your breasts between feedings.

Personal grooming items. Make sure you have the following: soap, hand lotion, comb, brush, mirror, toothbrush, toothpaste, lipstick, and emery board. You might also enjoy having some cologne with you.

Sanitary belt and pads for going home. Sometimes the hospital gives you some. Buy the giant size because you will still be discharging heavily.

A watch.

Something to read. Also a pen, stationery, and stamps. If you buy baby announcement cards ahead of time, the long days in the hospital are a marvelous time to get them written. This will mean one less thing you'll have to do during the *busy* days when you go home.

Some cash. Not a lot, but enough for newspapers, magazines, and other incidentals.

Fresh fruit or snack food (if your doctor okays it). The time between meals can sometimes seem long.

Different kinds of hospital rooms.

You may have a private room or you may be in a semi-private, which is usually two to four beds. Or you may be in a ward, which usually has more than four beds.

The private is most expensive, the ward is the least expensive. Many women like the two- to four-bed room because it gives them someone to talk to and to compare notes with.

The baby usually stays in the nursery and is brought to you frequently for feedings and cuddle time.

In rooming-in arrangements, the baby stays right with you in its crib, and you take care of it all during your hospital stay. This means more work for you, but also means you get to be close to your baby at all times and will know if it is crying. You can cuddle it when you want to, feed it when it needs it, and your husband can spend more time with the baby. Many doctors believe that rooming-in helps dispel the insecurity a baby can feel when it is in a central nursery away from mother.

How to cope with hospital red tape.

Most maternity services require preregistration so that your insurance data are on file.

It is helpful to have names ready, because a registrar will ask you the baby's name for the birth certificate. But, as noted previously, you can change your mind and add names, often merely by paying a small filing fee to the local department of health.

When you are going to check out, be sure to make arrangements the day before and have the doctor sign all the proper papers ahead of time so that you can be discharged promptly. Know when the discharge time is, because if you go past that time you can be charged for an extra day.

The patient's Bill of Rights.

Chances are everything is going to go smoothly and there will be no problems at all. But just in case some rare problem does occur, you should know about the patient's Bill of Rights recently formulated by the American Hospital Association. It is a part of a book given to all hospitals that cites the requirements for patient care and clearly spells out the following rights:

The patient has a right to physical privacy.

The patient has a right not to be used for teaching or research purposes except with his consent.

The patient has a right to know what is being done and why.

The patient has a right to know who is responsible for his case.

A patient should not be refused care because of race, creed, color, or national origin, or because of the source of payment of his bill.

If at any time you feel these rights have been transgressed, ask to see the social service representative or a person, found in some hospitals, called an ombudsman.

Classes in the hospital.

Most hospitals now give classes in how to hold a baby and bathe it, and in how to prepare formula. Other hospitals have added courses in contraceptive techniques, and some even have closed-circuit television with a variety of courses on health maintenance.

All of these courses are valuable and will help give you self-confidence.

Getting along with the hospital staff.

When you really need help, put on your light for a nurse. If it's an emergency, a real emergency, and no nurse comes, have your roommate call for one, or, if necessary, throw a bedpan out the door to get attention.

But don't expect the nurses to act like servants bringing you room service. Most things you can do yourself, and it is better that you do so, because the sooner you get up on your feet and move around, the better it is for you physically.

Sally M. told us her feelings of insecurity with the hospital nurses.

"Even in the hospital," she said, "although most of the nurses were very nice and cooperative, there were still a few who weren't. I was really insecure. I didn't know what to do. I didn't even feel like my baby was my child. Even though he was in the room with me, and I was allowed to take care of him and diaper him, I always hesitated. I felt that I needed the nurses' permission."

As in any group of people, some of the nurses are going to be warm and friendly, others are going to be cold and officious, or even crabby cranks. Ignore the cranks—that's *their* problem—and be friendly to the friendly ones.

Often when a nurse doesn't make any effort to help you it's because she assumes that you know how to handle a baby. It is so routine to her that she doesn't realize how strong that helpless, insecure feeling can be.

Try to keep a sense of perspective about it, realizing that you too in a few weeks will be an old hand at this and will be laughing at your insecurities. Meanwhile, meet the demands of the present by deciding which nurse you like the best and feel closest to, confess to her how absolutely stupid and insecure you feel, and ask her if she will spend some time to show you slowly and calmly how to diaper the baby, how to hold it, how to nurse it—whatever your immediate problem is. Be specific in your questions, since she hasn't the time to give you an entire course in baby care.

Getting along with your doctor.

The most important thing in relation to your doctor is to do what he says. An astounding number of people go to a doctor, listen, pay for the service, find out what to do to be healthy and live longer, and then completely ignore the advice.

The second most important thing is to talk to him. Tell him any fears you are having, any problems you have on your mind. We suggest that you keep a pad and pencil next to your bed to jot down questions as you think of them, ready to ask the next time he comes in.

If you want to know the medications you are taking, be sure to get the answers from your doctor or from the nurse who is administering the pill or injection. It is your right to know.

On checking out, check your bill.

To err is human, and to err and double err is about standard for a computer, so look over your bill carefully. It is not unheard of for girl babies to be charged for circumcision, and long distance phone calls to be charged when you didn't have a phone. Even when the bill will be paid by insurance, look it over. Any overcharges are reflected ultimately in increased premiums for everyone.

You will be expected to pay your bill before you leave, so be sure that your husband brings his checkbook with him when he comes to take you home.

How long will I be in the hospital?

Your length of stay will vary with the ease of your delivery or with any other procedures that were done.

The national average for hospital stay for delivery is three days. If you have a cesarean, hospitalization will last closer to one week.

In California, the Kaiser Permanente Medical Center has been keeping patients for only a day to a day and a half. They also have fathers present at delivery and offer rooming-in. During the time that the mother would ordinarily be in the hospital, a nurse makes daily visits to the home to check the mother and infant, do blood tests, and make out the birth certificate.

Home delivery.

Many women are now deciding to deliver their babies at home instead of in the hospital. It saves money, and they prefer the informality and the fact that they can take care of the baby immediately themselves.

Home delivery is fine for normal pregnancies and deliveries. You should not do it if you are a high-risk patient, that is, if you have diabetes, heart trouble, high blood pressure, have had complications during pregnancy, or had difficult deliveries in the past.

There are excellent home delivery services in many cities. Check with your doctor if you want to have your baby at home and follow his advice.

3

Going Home

Your doctor comes in with the big news. "Tomorrow you go home."

You grin, pleased. In fact, you're elated, and mentally you do a little jig, not quite up to doing it physically yet.

But there is also the shadow of insecurity slipping in again. This is it, girl. Tomorrow I go home and I'm a mother. It's all up to me.

You call your husband and tell him tomorrow is the big day. And then you lie back and wonder what the day will be like.

What's the check-out like? What should you have for the baby? What should you wear home? What if you drop the baby? What kind of papers have to be signed? What if they give you the wrong baby? What's the house look like? Do you have everything you need? What if you forget something important?

Let's take first things first.

You're not going to drop the baby because the nurse is going to carry it out all the way to the door.

It sounds silly, but how can I be sure my baby wasn't switched with someone else's?

While you are still in the delivery room, a nurse puts a bracelet on your arm and an identical bracelet on your baby's arm. The bracelet never comes off and is there for identification when your baby leaves the hospital with you.

Most hospitals also immediately footprint the new baby and place the mother's fingerprint on the same page. This assures that you are always matched.

The day before you check out.

Be sure to call the hospital business office or have your husband call to confirm the fact that your doctor has signed the proper papers for you to check out the next morning and that your bill will be ready. Also ask what the latest check-out time is so that you do not go beyond it.

Go over your list and make sure that you have everything together that you need for the baby and for yourself for the trip home. Call your husband and tell him the things that you still need him to bring in so he can write them down and bring them that night during visiting hours. The more organized you are beforehand, the less confusion there will be in the morning so that you can check out with dispatch.

If you tend to be disorganized or become nervous under stress, do your packing the evening before, giving one last look at your list to know that everything is there. Most people find, however, that it only takes about fifteen minutes to pack in the morning and prefer to do it then just before they get dressed.

If you haven't finished addressing your birth announcements, get them done so you don't have to worry about them at home.

If you are planning to have a maid, housekeeper, or relative help you with housework, call her and tell her when to come in.

Call the diaper service if you are going to have one and tell them when to start.

Read through your baby-care books one more time.

Resist the urge to call all your friends. You will want the first day or two at home undisturbed by friendly phone calls and visits.

What the baby needs for the trip home.

Don't overload with a lot of things you don't really need. Save Aunt Matilda's lace shawl and the hand-embroidered expensive import for another time. And don't overdress the baby—it doesn't need nearly as many sweaters and blankets as you think it does.

The following is an ample list, unless you are going a great distance that is apt to take more than an hour:

Three diapers (one on, one spare, and one to keep you from worrying)

Plastic panty

One undershirt

A gown or jumper suit

A bunting for most of the warmth

A hat

Socks

Booties

A blanket

What about formula?

Usually the hospital furnishes you with one day's supply of formula, or at least a bottle to get home on. And they will give you a bottle of sugar water to give to the baby if it frets on the way home, or if the trip home goes beyond his feeding time.

If they furnish a full day's supply of formula already made up, it is a marvelous help, since you don't have to worry about making it up the instant you arrive home. Those who breast-feed are obviously already ahead of the game.

What you need for the trip home.

Many women simply wear home the same maternity outfit that they came in with (sometimes on purpose; sometimes because they find on the morning of check-out that they can't fit into the dress or pants they packed to go home in!). If you wear a nonmaternity garment home, be sure it is one that is loose-fitting and large-waisted—something like what you were wearing at month three or four. Wear flat shoes for extra steadiness.

Also have ready your own sanitary belt with the largest (ask for hospital-size) pad available. Sometimes the hospital furnishes these, sometimes not.

If the drive home will be long, have your husband bring a pillow to make you more comfortable or to put on your lap to hold the baby.

What your husband should bring in.

The most important thing he can bring is a smile and a self-confident guiding hand.

Also be sure he brings the checkbook and any hospital insurance papers for taking care of the bill before you leave.

What baby needs to have ready at home.

Clothes that the baby needs are the following, depending on the season:

> Three to six dozen diapers (unless you have diaper service or will use disposable diapers)
> Six diaper pins
> A bar of soap to stick pins in
> Six cotton undershirts
> Three to six nightgowns
> Three to six stretch jumpsuits
> Six plastic panties, snap-style (not necessary with disposable diapers, which are covered with a moisture covering)
> Two sweaters
> Six pairs of socks
> Two booties
> One bunting
> One knitted cap
> Six light cotton receiving blankets
> Twelve bibs
> Disposable diapers
> Diaper liners

Bath items, in addition to the small tub, should include the following:

Four washcloths
Four towels
Cotton swabs with flexible plastic sticks
Cotton
Baby oil
Baby fingernail scissors
Soap
Rectal thermometer
Baby no-tear shampoo
Vaseline

Other equipment and miscellaneous items that the baby needs will include the following:

Baby carriage, with sheets or pillowcases to cover pad
Sterilizer
Twelve 8-ounce bottles
Six 4-ounce bottles
Twenty-four nipples
Four pacifiers
Vaporizer (He is going to have a bad cold sooner or later, so you may as well buy it now instead of rushing out later.)
Baby vitamins (Your pediatrician will specify kind.)
Car bed

What you need ready at home for yourself.

You should buy things ahead of time for yourself also.

You should have several good nursing bras, with an ample supply of pads for inserting into the cups.

You should have several boxes of large-sized sanitary pads and a wide sanitary belt. (The wide kind is more comfortable when you must wear it for a long time. Buy two so you can launder.)

Have several extra pairs of pajamas or nightgowns because you may be needing more than usual for the first few days. With your vaginal discharge, your milk coming in, plus the baby burping on you, you will need frequent changes.

And have plenty of comfortable clothes ready to wear with buttons sewn on and ironed so you can have something to get into when you put all those maternity tents away.

Some doctors recommend that maternity girdles be worn in the postpartum period. They are not necessary but you certainly may use them if they make you feel more comfortable.

You might also want to make out a grocery list so that your husband can do some shopping and have the pantry and refrigerator well stocked when you get home.

Advice about the nursery.

The baby's room will be his first home, so you want it to be just right. But keep it simple.

Here is a list of things you will wish to consider for the nursery to be ready when you and the baby come home:

A room to himself if possible (freshly scrubbed, or painted with nonlead paint in bright colors)

A bassinet (or basket or crib made smaller with crib bumpers)

Knit fitted sheets (no top sheet needed)

No pillow

A blanket

A table (or other surface for dressing the baby on)

A bathinette, if you want to be fancy, a plastic bathtub if you want to be simple

Storage space (either a chest of drawers or shelves, for clothes, diapers, and supplies)

A diaper pail

A plastic pail or hamper for dirty clothes

Bright pictures or sculptured forms to catch baby's eye

A crib mobile for baby to jiggle and study

A rocking chair for cuddling and feeding times

4

Attitudes
Toward Yourself

Karen H. was a public relations consultant, an intelligent girl who had looked forward to her pregnancy. She had shopped for her baby's wardrobe with enthusiasm and had planned every detail of the baby's room. It had bright colors, hanging mobiles so the baby would have things to look at for stimulation, and even an aquarium of tropical fish for a bright accent.

Three weeks after she was home from the hospital she sat in her rocking chair at two in the morning, tired and depressed. The baby was screaming. She couldn't get him to take milk or burp up a bubble. She tried everything—rocked him, burped him, put him over her knee, patted and massaged him, and checked for dirty diapers or an open safety pin. The baby cried on and on.

"Suddenly, I could hardly believe it," Karen said. "I looked at that kid and hated him with all my heart. 'Why do you make me feel so helpless? What did I ever do to make you treat me this way? Where's your appreciation for all we've done for you?'

"I knew he couldn't answer. I knew he couldn't help it. But it didn't matter. I actually hated him!

"And those stupid fish kept swimming back and forth, back and forth. And I hated *them!* I could have picked up both them and the baby in that moment and thrown them out the window!

"Then, immediately, I felt guilty for the hatred. I looked at that tiny hunk of helplessness. And I hated *myself!*"

Does it sound shocking? Or, if you're a new mother, does it sound only too familiar?

Nearly every mother we spoke to had similar feelings toward her baby at some time during the postpartum period. But since they didn't know other women had times when they felt the same way, they felt like real beasts, were ashamed and guilty, and hid their feelings.

"I suddenly one day just didn't want my child. I just wanted to be happy and carefree like I was before."

Agnes S., happily married for three years before her pregnancy, and still happily married, we might add, said, "Nobody tells you much about coming home with a new baby. I was not aware of the constancy of it, that the baby is *always* there."

Rita H. said the feeling of desperation struck her about the fourth week. "I wasn't expecting it because I've looked after a lot of young children," she said. "But I felt totally lost suddenly after I got home. This was *my* child. *I* was completely responsible for it. I just wasn't prepared for the great emotion that hit me."

How many women have these difficulties?

When we asked women about these feelings of hostility and anger, almost every single mother said she had such feelings at some time. All of the women said that they were not prepared. They said that they were happy when they came home and then were totally surprised when these different feelings came upon them and they had to cope with them.

What can you do about this feeling?

The first thing you should do is not feel guilty about it. Know that other women go through the same thing. You are not alone. You are not some sort of monster. The feelings are normal. And the feelings will pass.

Discuss your emotions with your husband. He may be having some ambivalent feelings also. Talking them out together can be a tremendous relief to both of you and make everything easier to handle, instead of letting tensions build up because you bottle up the feelings and worry about them.

Then a good thing for you and your husband to do is get a baby-sitter and get out. Go to a restaurant for dinner. Don't worry about leaving your baby for a short time with a responsible sitter. Get out on your own again. Redefine your life together.

What are baby blues?

This is another name for what doctors call postpartum depression. Not every woman gets them. Dorothy said she never did go through a period of depression. "My husband kept saying I was going to get depressed. My mother said I was going to be depressed. My doctor said I should expect it. But I just never did."

Some women go through a short period of the blues. Others really have severe problems. In fact, not too many years ago psychosis was common after delivery. In many states the board of health required iron bars on all windows of the obstetrics floors to prevent suicide.

The typical reaction in postpartum depression is to suddenly feel that everything is wrong, that you just can't cope: you feel completely tired and worn out, and you just want to sit down and cry. And often you will. Sometimes about something in particular. Sometimes about nothing at all. You just feel like you need a good cry.

There are less typical ways of showing the depression. Outbursts of anger of inappropriate degree or inappropriate degrees of concern about minute details are often signs of depression. For example, one new mother became obsessed with the cleanliness of her home on returning from the hospital. She began to spend hours cleaning corners and moldings and polishing floors as a means of denying and not facing her inner feelings of sadness and mourning.

Sometimes the blues will hit a new mother right in the hospital on the second or third day, but more often it hits at home. Sometimes it will double-barrel you both in the hospital and at home.

Some doctors believe that postpartum depression is completely caused by emotional tensions. But the evidence points strongly to the fact that in most women it is a combination of the effects of hormonal changes after pregnancy and the emotional changes and the new intensifications that motherhood brings.

Both estrogen and progesterone hormone levels that were high during pregnancy, now that the hormones are unneeded, drop precipitously after delivery.

The new mother may report hot flashes on the second or third postpartum day identical to the hot flashes of the menopause. These probably reflect an adjustment to the falling estrogen levels.

A large amount of urine will be formed during these few days, since body fluid is no longer retained as it was during pregnancy. It is a further physical sign of the hormonal changes.

When the menopausal woman is given estrogen-replacement therapy, she usually reports a sense of "well-being." The postpartum mother is losing estrogen and reports a loss of "well-being," in other words, a feeling of depression.

What can I do for the baby blues?

Again, remember that "this too shall pass." The depression usually occurs in waves, and the frequency of the waves of sadness gets less as the first weeks pass. And then you'll be feeling back on top of the world again, able to cope with ease, able to look at the problems that now seem like insurmountable mountains and skim over them like the molehills they really are.

Look at the baby blues as a warning sign, however. A

warning that you need to devote more time to yourself and to your relationship with your husband.

Change your environment and increase your external stimuli. Make yourself get away. During the day, let the washing or ironing or whatever go, take your baby for a walk. Or while the baby is sleeping, go for a short walk yourself. Line up a baby-sitter for the evening. You and your husband get dressed up like you used to, go out, and talk about something besides the baby. It's like taking yourself out of mourning. And it really seems to work. When you get to that restaurant, you suddenly begin to realize that it is not so bad after all.

There's something about being responsible all day long without a break. You are the person in charge. It's a full-time job, plus. You are actually confined, tied down, committed.

Getting out to that restaurant proves that you are not really as confined as you thought you were. It is physical proof of an independence you tend to forget that you have.

In fact, it's a good idea to line up your baby-sitter regularly, say, every Friday night, so that it is not too difficult to make arrangements to get you away from the baby. If you cannot afford a sitter that often, try to work it out with a relative, or trade off with a friend who also would like to have a sitter. You can sit for her on a different night.

If the disturbing feelings persist and you really can't seem to shake the depression, talk to your obstetrician and discuss your feelings with him. If you need professional help, you should get it so that you have the best situation for yourself and are best able to take care of your child. If your obstetrician does not refer you to someone who can provide such help, call your local family service agency, describe your situation, and ask if you can be seen quickly.

How can I tell if my depression is excessive?

The depression is excessive if it prevents you from meeting your basic responsibilities. These are responsibilities to yourself, to your baby, and to your husband.

The responsibilities to the baby are very basic. You should be able to provide food and shelter and love.

Your responsibility to yourself is the maintenance of good hygiene and cleanliness and an adequate diet.

And to your husband you should be able to keep open lines of communication about your feelings.

Mourning the loss of what you used to be.

One can look upon postpartum depression as a feeling of mourning for the person that you used to be. Suddenly you feel that you have lost the carefree and independent spirit that you were. The obvious dependence of the baby makes you feel dependent yourself, because as you try to relate to the child, you must go through a period of identification with the child, almost like being the baby yourself. This, coupled with the feeling of responsibility, gives you a sense of loss for who you were.

We can objectively and intellectually discuss the fact that you are really the same person, carefree and independent, with the baby added. We can say that the baby and its responsibilities are to be integrated or added to your original personality, and it makes sense—until you actually feel the mourning or depression.

The one way to deal with it is to mechanically assert that you are the same person that you were. A good way to do this is to get away from the baby and enjoy and engage in some activity that you've enjoyed before. Like going out with your husband and showing yourself that you can still relate now as you did before. You can still talk about topics other than the baby; you can still enjoy aspects of life that you enjoyed before the baby was born. Your spirit is indeed the same, with something added.

Tired mother's syndrome.

Taking care of the baby around the clock can wear anybody out. The constant child care plus housework can be both physically and psychologically fatiguing and can soon lead to utter exhaustion—the tired mother's syndrome. This in turn can be the major factor in the postpartum depression. It's hard to be happy when you can hardly hold your head up because of exhaustion.

Take frequent rests. Take your vitamins and iron pills. Get out at least once a week. You have a duty to your husband and to your family to do the most important thing—to take care of yourself.

What about taking baby with you when you go out?

You should go out once in a while without the baby, even if you don't want to or if it is difficult. It is absolutely necessary for your own emotional well-being, for the closeness of feelings between you and your husband, and even best for the baby, so that it doesn't become completely dependent on being with you.

But there is nothing wrong with taking the baby with you sometimes too. It's good for a baby to be exposed to different environments, and it's a great together feeling to go traipsing off as mother and baby or as a family unit of father, mother, and child.

The baby couldn't care less about what it is seeing at this point. The zoo is no different from a walk in the park. But the fresh air and being together and being around the stimulation of other people and things is great for everybody. In fact, one thing that will often soothe a cranky baby is the lulling rhythm of a car ride, a ride in a buggy, or even a boat ride. Scott Linde, at age three months, went out almost every summer evening for a gentle, careful boat ride around the shore for twenty minutes or so. It worked wonders for quieting prolonged crying.

Travel as lightly as you can so that the trip can be spontaneous and not too much trouble. Just have plenty of disposable diapers along, a bottle of milk, and some dry clothes. Then, with a carefree outlook, go have a lark together, whether it's a trip to the store or a visit to a friend.

One tiny note of caution: If you visit a friend's house and put the baby on the bed for a nap, be sure to surround it with large pillows or other barricade. Even the smallest new baby can squirm enough to make it to the side of the bed in what seems like no time. And be sure to put a towel or a diaper under the baby. The best diapers leak, and frequently an inadvertent burp can occur.

What about nursing in public?

It depends on how you feel about it. If it makes you uncomfortable, then do not nurse in public, do it privately. If you are at a friend's house, you can easily excuse yourself and go into the next room.

If you are relaxed about it, and it does not make you uncomfortable, then go ahead. In most areas now, nursing in public is considered permissible. Just be unobtrusive and turn your back slightly and you will be mostly hidden. If the milk does not come readily, it means that it is not right for you, no matter how much you think it is all right on the conscious level.

Does it ever really change?

Yes, it truly does.

Heidi's experience was typical. "The first week was very hard, but the second week you're less tired. And every week after that gets a little better. You become confident that the baby is going to sleep and eat and do everything normally, despite all your fears and misgivings. And suddenly everything begins to fall in place, and you start feeling good about life and about yourself again."

Motherhood is not a contest.

One thing to remember as you start out in your new role is that you are not trying to prove anything to anybody. Not even yourself. This isn't a contest. There is no one way to be a parent and raise a child. There is no one attitude to have. There is no absolutely right way. There are many styles of being a parent and raising a child. It's a matter of finding the style that's right for you.

Don't try to be the All-American Perfect Mother. You won't be perfect, no matter how great you are. You may as well relax as you discover some mistakes you have made. Of course, you are going to do the best things you possibly can for your child. Of course, you are going to see that it is taken care of and cuddled and loved. But don't be uptight and on stage every minute. The Superperfect 100-Percent-Mistake-Proof Mother hasn't been created yet.

You will soon find that most of the time you have a delicacy of feeling and a feeling of accomplishment. You will have a sense of being comfortable with your baby and yourself, of enjoying yourself in this new experience, and of enjoying the baby.

How to relieve tension.

The first step to relieving tension is to recognize when you have it.

There are several signs: butterflies in the stomach, tight neck and jaw muscles, sweating palms, irritability, moving too brusquely with muscles tight, tightened voice. Or you may find your chin jutted out, your shoulders hunched, your spine rigid, your forehead tight with a headache coming on.

Many people, once they learn to recognize these symptoms in themselves, can turn them off fairly simply. They breathe deeply and slowly, one by one let their muscles relax, and mentally stroke themselves on the head as they tell themselves soothingly to relax.

How can I learn to relax?

It's a gradual adjustment. At first you are worrying about many details. Everything is a hurdle. Is the baby normal? Am I doing everything right? Is the bath right? the formula right? If the baby cries, you react too fast.

You're on edge, you're uptight, and you're trying too hard.

There are several things you can do. One is to talk to yourself, simply make the decision that you are consciously going to be more relaxed.

Second is to definitely schedule time for naps and relaxation for yourself. Sometimes it's not so much tension as fatigue that makes the new mother uncomfortable. Schedule relaxation time for yourself and for your husband. The time is there. You simply must arrange for it.

Third, consciously practice relaxation exercises. Sometimes simply putting on some soothing music and training yourself to move more slowly will do it. When you feel yourself getting tense, breathe deeply several times and consciously let your muscles go. Or you may want to do your relaxing on a more formalized basis. Practice progressive relaxation exercises. Lie down and drift while counting from one to ten, or imagine a series of numbers painted langorously in the sky, or picture yourself drifting slowly on a cloud, or swimming through soft waves on a balmy, blue sea. You may want to buy a book on beginning yoga and practice the relaxation exercises of the yoga masters. One of the simplest exercises is to lie on your back completely relaxed. Imagine you are a sponge, arms limp and away from the body, shoulders relaxed, legs apart and loose. Press your neck and back into the bed. Close your eyes, breathe deeply through your nose, relax each part of your body, beginning with your toes, working up to your fingers, wrists, and arms, right up your neck; relax your facial muscles and even your scalp muscles.

Yoga exercises or other methods of transcendental relaxation work for many people, enabling them to experience moments of internal retreat and to relax at will. The deep breathing and mind control exercises can be effective as tranquilizers, helping your body and mind function like a running stream—smooth and flowing.

Learn abdominal breathing. This low, quiet breathing will calm emotions and induce restful sleep. It can be done lying flat on your back, with knees bent and feet drawn to the buttocks, or sitting in a chair. Place one hand on your abdomen and one on your chest, so you can feel that you are breathing with the abdomen alone, not with the chest. Inhale deeply through the nostrils and expand the abdomen without pulling the air up to the chest. Keep your shoulders and chest relaxed. Exhale slowly through the nostrils while pulling the abdomen to the back of the spine. Practice this at the end of your other exercises when you go to bed at night or as often as you wish during the day when you want to relax.

Rachel Carr in her book *Yoga for All Ages* describes these breathing exercises as excellent not only for relaxation but also for overcoming depression.

"Whenever dark thoughts enter your mind," says Carr, "take a deep breath and draw into your body the forces of energy, strength, and tranquility. Then exhale and slowly empty all negative thoughts like a gently moving current of water until the good thoughts remain. . . . Be conscious of your deep, quiet breathing. . . . Let your mind rest in a climate of serenity. Think of yourself as a vast ocean. The waves that rise and fall are your thoughts, thoughts generated by external elements, like waves moved by soft winds and deep currents. Don't cling to them. They are only fleeting and will change like the waves of the ocean."

What is the meditation state?

Technically, it's a state of alpha, your brain putting out alpha waves as it does in the first moments of falling asleep. It's a quiet state of inner reflection. To experience meditation, allow at least twenty minutes of relaxed time.

As you did in the relaxation exercises, take deep, slow, long breaths. Feel a calming influence coming over and into your body. With eyes closed, breathe rhythmically and quietly. Let your muscles relax, let your mind blank to nothing . . . drifting. Don't work at it, just let it happen. Let your mind wander as it wishes. Observe it, but don't try to control it. Now and then you will enter into brief deeper interludes of retreat. If you are completely relaxed, you are experiencing meditation. If you have access to biofeedback apparatus, you can know if you are in the alpha state because of the steady hum of the machine.

I feel so unattractive.

You may feel unappealing and homely. Your abdomen is not yet flat and your hair may feel limp. And you may be discouraged with having to wear sanitary pads for such a long time.

The answer is obvious. It is time for a shower, time to wash your hair, or have a new cut, have a manicure, do some exercise, and put on fresh clothes.

The feeling of being unattractive is usually a reflection of some underlying feelings of depression. It is certainly a time to follow basic grooming rules and a time for some introspective analysis.

Somehow fixing it all up on the outside seems to help fix it up on the inside, too. And there isn't a woman in the world who doesn't feel a little bit like a new women with a new outlook on life when she looks good.

Something terrible is going to happen.

Many women who are happily married, comfortably settled in their homes, their days serene and routine, come to the doctor faltering and unsure. "I can't explain it. I'm just afraid something terrible is going to happen to me."

They are doing exactly what they have always dreamed of doing and yet they have anxiety, a feeling of impending doom.

Dr. Robert Seidenberg, a psychiatrist in Syracuse, New York, has talked to many such women and feels the women sense the danger of their lives being too secure and set. He calls the syndrome "the trauma of eventlessness."

"It's not what actually happens to these women, but what *fails* to happen to them," he says. "People need an element of challenge and change and risk in their lives, and it is these elements that are so often denied to the housewife."

This can be a problem after pregnancy also. The psychological workings of becoming nonpregnant are not necessarily easy. You are no longer the center of attention, you see your life seemingly mapped out for years with you as your child's servant, you may have stopped working and feel that void, and you are lonely being home all day with no one to talk to. No feedback, no appreciation, no conversation.

Right now there's not too much you can do except to see that your days are filled with some things besides baby. Read a book that makes you think, listen to music that excites you, make sure you get out frequently. Plan your return to your career, even if only on a part-time basis. And once the postpartum period is over, be sure your life doesn't become stale, that you make it as exciting for the three of you as it was before for the two of you—or even more so.

If you want to work.

Whether to mix career and motherhood is a big question for many new mothers and only you can answer for yourself. It can be done either way—stay home and resume your carcer later, or get someone to take care of the baby and go back to work right away.

Some say, "It's not the amount of time you spend with your children, but the quality that counts."

Others say nothing substitutes for being there when your child gets sick or hurts himself, that you can't be a mother by telephone, that the mother-substitute won't do things just the way you want her to. Also a child's needs are unpredictable—he can't program first words and other triumphs or worries or accidents just between 5:00 P.M. and bedtime.

The two hardest things to manage are organization of time —it often seems as if there aren't enough hours to get everything done—and fatigue. You not only run out of time, but you may also run out of energy.

The other difficulty, of course, is finding the right person to take care of the baby. Let us hope and fight to get more day-care centers and Head Start programs to help solve the problem.

It is important not to be pressured either way. If you want to stay home and be with your baby—do it. If you resent staying home and want to be at work—do that. Or if you're lucky, perhaps you can free-lance or work part time at your job and have the benefits both ways. Or take off for the first important years, then go back to your job.

It's important for you to decide what will make you happiest, give you the most satisfaction, and what is going to be best for your baby. Then confidently be the stay-at-home mother *or* be the working mother. Think it through carefully. Make your own decision. If you think later that you erred, then be willing to change.

Whatever you choose—to stay at home or to work—enjoy the commitment and be prepared to reevaluate it on a regular basis.

Care of the baby if you work.

A mother who must leave her baby in someone else's care during the whole day, or some part of it, feels happier about it if the baby is handled in much the same way that she would handle it.

The fewer differences there are in a baby's care, the more comfortable baby feels. If the person caring for the baby during the week holds it and rocks it to sleep, the baby will probably cry if it is not rocked when its mother takes over during the weekend.

Written instructions to your stand-in about important details of baby's care will be helpful.

When you find the person who will take care of your baby, whether it is a relative, friend, or someone you hire, make sure it is someone who will stay on the job. It is actually a more difficult adjustment for you than for the baby to have frequent changes in the person who cares for it.

Supervise the sitter before you leave the baby alone with that person.

Your main concern is that the person who cares for the baby be warm and motherly and really enjoy babies.

Try not to be jealous of the affection baby comes to feel for its part-time "mother." Instead, be glad your baby can enjoy such a good relationship.

If you should have to board your baby away from home, be sure the home you pick meets your standards.

What are the basic rules for being a happy new mother?

There are probably three basic rules you should remember.

1. No matter what feelings you are having, remember that others have them too. You are not alone. And you have no reason to feel guilty or scared about your feelings. They are legitimate and meaningful.

2. Remember that the baby is not you. It is an extension of you, but you are not it, and it is not you. Your baby is an individual, separate person.

3. You need to realize that you are the same person you were before the baby was born. Your life can still be much the same. You can still relate to your husband in the same way and to your parents and friends in the same way, still do the things you like to do. Everything that we experience of course changes us in a subtle way, adds on to the fiber of what we are. But underneath we are still the same person.

Even as a mother, you are the same person that you used to be, and your husband is the same person he used to be.

If you can understand these three guidelines, then you can cope successfully no matter how threatening things seem.

When do you get the mother instinct?

"I never had any trouble being a girl. I liked the idea of being pregnant, looked forward to having the baby, was ecstatic in fact. But somehow I just didn't feel like a *mother.*"

"I would sit there and look at this little hunk of humanity, and I loved it in a neutral sort of way like you love any tiny baby. But it didn't feel like *mine.* I didn't have that red, white, and blue, flags-waving, bells-ringing, rush-of-maternal-glow that I felt I should have."

"It scared me. Really. I still felt like a little peanut who used to run home from school and play baseball, who used to sit on the seashore and wonder what it would be like to be grown up and be a wife and a mother and be doing things in the world instead of getting ready to be doing them. And here all of a sudden, I *was* grown up, I was really doing all of it. But I didn't *feel* anything."

It was a group of new mothers talking again. Most of these women had had their babies six months to a year before, so that they had a chance to look back on the experience with some perspective. The one thing they found was a sense of relief in knowing that other women had had the same feelings, the same doubts.

"I took care of my baby all right," one woman said. "But I just never felt like a mother." Then, talking about our sessions together, she said, "I didn't realize that it was okay to be that way until right now."

Another woman said, "You know, you can't fall in love with a baby just because it is born and is handed to you. The first time I really loved him was when he got his shot when he was six weeks old. I felt he really needed me then."

Another summed it up well for all of them. "I believe that maternal love grows. It is not an instant emotion. Like falling in love with your husband is not an instant emotion. You've been practicing it all your life up until the time you meet whomever you fall in love with. And even then it may come on very gradually. You find more and more in him to love as time goes by."

And indeed, most of the women said that it was at about three months that they really learned to love their babies completely. And they also found that while "maternal instinct" seemed fleeting and elusive with their first baby, it came in a rush with the second.

If all of this sounds strange to you, if maternal love came on strong and instantaneously with you, then great. You're already ahead of the game. On the other hand, if you're a woman who feels more like a sister than a mother, don't fret, you will end up feeling like a mother soon. We'll talk more about this in the next chapter.

5

How You Feel
About Your Baby

The day you leave the hospital, you stand poised at the hospital door, the nurse hands you your baby, and with your husband standing beside you, you feel that you make up the Happy Ideal Perfect American Family. The sun's rays glimmer across the blue sky, you can almost hear the music rising in a crescendo as you step—the Perfect Threesome—toward your car.

But the Hollywood-like fantasy blurs and fades into a more serious reality. That reality may dawn when the baby begins to cry unexpectedly, or when you realize that the diaper should be changed when your car is stopped by traffic.

And the new image blurs more at home when you begin to feel fatigue with some of your new jobs, as you realize that you are not immediately as efficient as you would like to be, and when you see that a baby doesn't always do what the book says it should.

Welcome to reality! The trying times as well as the good times make up what becoming a family is really all about.

There will be enough marvelous moments to set off the bad ones. Moments when you gaze at your newborn baby and think again of the miracle of its growing from two tiny cells to the billions of cells that make a human being with a life of its own. Moments when you see your child asleep with complete bliss and innocence upon its face, knowing that everything in the world that it depends on, you are responsible for. Moments when your eyes meet and the baby recognizes you. The moment the baby first hesitantly smiles at you. Moments when its tiny hands, amazingly strong, grip yours, and you picture these hands when your baby is grown up, when these hands will be those of a grown man or woman building bridges, playing a piano, caressing another human in love.

You think how hands are so important—they can be strong and competent and helping others, like you want your child's to be. Or they can be weak and fumbling or greedy hands.

The world's future will soon be in the hands of today's children. And those children will be what we make them. They come to us as clay, dependent upon what we provide and what we teach. They leave us as men and women, the next generation, as we have molded them.

When my baby cries, what am I doing wrong?

Probably nothing. If you've looked for all the usual things, like overheated milk, a need to burp, diaper rash or other hurts, or the baby being too hot or too cold or wanting to be turned over to another position or its having an earache or getting a new tooth, then probably the baby has a stomachache or something else, something that is unavoidable. All you can do at this point is sympathize, cuddle the baby if it seems to help, and if it doesn't, put it down and hope it falls asleep soon.

The important thing is not to feel inadequate because of the crying. It's usually not your fault.

As a matter of fact, two psychiatrists at the University of

Colorado, Drs. Robert N. Emde and Robert J. Harmon, studied a group of babies from birth to one year and found that occasionally, in their exact words, "All the babies fussed without apparent physical cause, and their crying seemed to have nothing to do with the quality of the mothering."

Your baby needs nourishment, a safe, comfortable place to sleep, and clothing to keep it cozy and warm. It needs to have its excretions removed and its body kept relatively clean. It needs to be burped if it swallows air. It needs love. It needs special help for diaper rash, a stuffy nose, an earache or a new tooth, or other problems.

If you have done everything you can think of, then you will have to decide whether the fussy baby is bored and needs attention, has an ache and needs to be comforted, or is overtired and simply needs to be left alone for a short time to cry and fall asleep.

How can I tell what his cry means?

When your baby cries, how do you know if it is from hunger, pain, diaper rash, or just a desire for some pleasurable interaction with another human being?

At first you don't. It is sheer trial and error. Later you begin to sense the difference. It's amazing how a "hungry" cry soon sounds different from an "I'm-in-pain" cry.

At first you may have to consider a number of possibilities until you can tell one kind of cry from another.

The U.S. Public Health Service recommends the following.

1. All babies cannot be expected to fall asleep at once after they are fed. Wait for five to ten minutes to see if it won't settle down. If the crying shows no signs of letting up, pat the baby for a while right in the crib. If that doesn't calm the baby, pick it up and hold and soothe it. Usually by this time the baby is wet again, or has had a bowel movement, so it won't hurt to change the diaper.

2. If a baby seems to go sound asleep after a feeding, but then wakes up and cries within a half hour, a good guess is that it didn't get all the air bubbles up and is having gas

pains. Burp the baby again. Don't try to put it down again too soon.

3. If it has been two hours or more since the baby was last fed, it may be hungry. If it is hungry, it will not be contented by being held, but will squirm and search from side to side with its mouth, hunting for the nipple, or will act restless. This hunting action is called "rooting."

4. A few babies seem to be uncomfortable when they are wet and settle down to sleep quickly when they are changed. Some quiet down after they have had an ounce or two of warm water. Other possibilities are that the baby may be too warm or too cold. These are easy things to check on.

5. Many babies fall asleep readily when they are rocked, taken for a ride in a car, or wheeled about in a carriage. A fussy baby often quiets down and sleeps when its father or mother rocks it or walks with the baby a little while. Some babies are soothed to sleep by a loud-ticking clock or by the hum of an electric fan.

Keep in mind that a little crying (five or ten minutes several times a day) is to be expected and does no harm. But *when there is a great deal of crying, you need your doctor's help.*

That so-called maternal touch.

Much of the early awkwardness with our feelings toward ourselves as mothers is mirrored in the way we touch our infants. In fact, how we touch our new babies shows that a sudden instinct of motherly love is not universal, that most motherly love starts tentatively.

Reva Rubin writes in *Nursing Outlook* that new mothers on the maternity ward do not impulsively enfold their new infants.

"Feelings of maternal love are not endowed, but are acquired over time," says Rubin, and how the new mother touches her infant affects this.

"In the maternity wards, there is a definite progression and an orderly sequence in the nature and amount of contact a mother makes with her child. At first only her fingertips are involved, then her hands (including her palms) and then, much later, her whole arms."

The initial contacts made by the mother to her child are exploratory, Rubin says. At this point, the mother will usually run one fingertip over the baby's hair, rather than a hand, to discover that his hair is silky. "She will trace his profile and contours with her fingertip. If she turns his head towards food, she uses fingertips; if she has to support his head as in bathing, she'll use the index finger and thumb (no palm), and if she has to turn him, she seems to get some ends of him with her fingertips. She does use her arms and her hands, but usually to passively receive him, her arms are not active participators in touch at this stage. She carries the baby in her arm as though it were a bouquet of flowers and her arm is held so stiffly that she becomes fatigued."

In maternal touch, the fingertip stage precedes that of commitment, Rubin says. Commitment seems to await some response from the infant.

The new mother is very vulnerable at this time to signs of rejection as well as responsiveness, she says. But if the young mother has an essentially strong ego, she will search out signs of response for a progressive relationship.

The next stage of maternal touch arrives gradually, Rubin says. "The whole hand is used for maximal contact with the infant's body. Her hand on his back will be in full contact in every available surface of her palm and fingers. Her hands are relaxed and comfortable, representing how she feels about herself in her relationship with him. Her security in herself is transmitted, through touch, to him, and his responsiveness to her firm, comforting touch feeds back into her own well-being.

"We see only the beginnings of this stage in the maternity wards. Somewhere between the third and fifth days postpartally, we see her stroke her baby's head with her whole hand, cupped, in place of a fingertip. . . . Her arms and shoulders get progressively more relaxed and the distance between her body and that of the baby becomes shorter."

Interestingly, it was found that mothers who had been touched frequently by a ministering person in labor and delivery or in the postpartum period used their own hands more effectively with their babies and progressed more quickly from one stage to another.

How often should I pick the baby up?

Just as often as you want. Don't worry about spoiling it. Pick it up, love it, talk to it as you walk by. The baby may be crying because it's bored.

The more stimulation and enrichment of all kinds your child gets, the better off it is. Give it not only the stimulation of being held and talked to, but provide it fascinating things to look at and things to touch and grasp. Research has shown that environmental stimuli will speed up baby development markedly in the first six months of life.

Holding your baby often and long can make you feel closer to it and can help you relate to it better. A famous study by Drs. Klaus and Kennell in Cleveland showed the importance of this, even in the very beginning in the hospital. One group of mothers and infants were managed in the usual way after delivery. A second group of mothers were given their infants to hold for an entire hour within minutes after delivery and also held their infants for a total of five hours a day throughout the hospital stay. One month later the mothers in the experimental group showed more interest in their babies and spent more face-to-face time with them.

What can I do to hurry mother instinct?

Let yourself relax with the baby. As you relax, your actions become gentler, smoother, more soothing. Then the baby becomes relaxed too.

Hold your baby and cuddle it. It's not as fragile as you think. Touch it, explore its body with your hands, feel the marvelously smooth skin and downy peach-fuzz hair. Talk to it, sing sweet or silly lullabies even if you've never sung to anyone before.

As one woman said, "What really did it for me was to hold my baby, talk to it about the wonderful life it was going to have, and let myself wallow in a puddle of sentimentality that made me feel completely happy."

Breast-feeding in a rocking chair is a marvelous way of

getting to know your baby. There are few things in life more satisfying than when the baby nestles in your arms, roots for the breast, then settles back in sheer luxury while you nurse it and contentedly rock.

Will I be a slave to my baby?

At first, with your new baby a totally helpless creature, you may feel like a slave—and completely unappreciated. Helping a baby is not a give-and-take relationship like your marriage. It's all *you* give and *it* takes.

You must see that you do not become completely centered around the baby, do not become a slave to it. Leave time for yourself and your husband.

Your baby will soon be expanding its world, taking in many things outside the now confining crib. You too must once more expand your world and your horizons.

And soon your relationship with your child will not be all give. It will give you something in return—love, trust, and the satisfaction you will feel in seeing the baby grow into a healthy, happy person.

I resent being 100-percent mother.

Things will ease up. None of the chores in taking care of the baby are really difficult—it's just that there are so many of them, and they are all new. In addition, you're still just getting your strength back.

Everything takes time at first because you are learning. As soon as things get to be routine, they'll go faster than you think.

Meanwhile, don't resent what you do so much, but try to do it with tenderness and affection. You can resent and swear all you want at the laundry and vacuuming, but it's important that you feel good when you feed and bathe and dress the baby.

I keep dreaming the baby is going to die.

Not uncommon. Shirley used to wake up often in a cold sweat because of a recurring nightmare that she was nursing the baby in the middle of the night and, exhausted and sleepy, fell asleep on top of the baby and smothered it to death.

Sherry said she worried a lot and often found herself overcome with terror that her baby was going to die, and there would be no one there to help it. "I would go through this weird thing," she said. "Being tired and mad and finding myself wishing the baby were dead and then going in to check it to make sure it wasn't. You feel so guilty and it makes you worry more."

Crib deaths—those strange, unexplained deaths that occur while a baby sleeps—receive publicity because they are mysterious. Doctors simply cannot find the cause despite much research and study. But they are very rare and need not be of concern.

If you have some premonition that something is happening, of course, go in and check the baby. And naturally you check it when you come home from being out at dinner or the theater, and last thing before you go to bed. But don't sit around nervously worrying about the baby every minute.

Avoiding accidents.

The most important thing to do is to protect your new baby from falling. Falls, plus fire, cause more injury to babies than any other accidents.

If you are visiting, don't put the baby on a bed unattended for a nap, free to squirm to the edge. Surround it with pillows or other soft barriers.

If you're changing diapers or giving baby a bath, don't leave it for a second! Not even to walk ten feet if you forgot something or to answer the phone. Take an extra instant to wrap the baby in a towel and carry it with you. That way, if your phone is next to the bed, you can dress the baby while you sit on your bed, which is easier than doing it standing up anyway.

Feeling jealous of the baby.

Jealous of your own baby? That sounds silly when you hear it, and even seems silly while it's happening. But it does happen. Your house was your domain and suddenly you have to share it with the baby. Your husband showered all his attentions on you, now you have to share him with the baby.

Sometimes the same thing will happen even with a new dog that a couple has. Haven't you ever seen your mate playing happily with a dog, romping, cuddling, laughing, and felt a sudden pang of jealousy for the attention, even though you knew it was absolutely insane? These same feelings can happen with the baby, but stronger, deeper. All you can do is recognize them, laugh at them, and remind yourself that love is not something that has to be divided among the people who share it, but the more it is spread, the more it multiplies and grows as your family and experience grows.

How do I know my child is developing properly?

No two children are alike. Perfectly normal, healthy children will walk and talk at different times. Naturally you will be proud of every accomplishment, but appreciate your child for what it is. Don't try to push development.

Here are some general guidelines to development from the American Medical Association.

One month—Can lift chin off table.

Two months—Can lift chest off table.

Three months—Reaches for objects but without success.

Four months—Can sit with support.

Five months—Can sit on lap and can grasp small objects.

Six months—Can sit in high chair and grasp a dangling object.

Seven months—Can sit alone.

Eight months—Can stand with help.

Nine months—Can stand by holding onto a piece of furniture.

Ten months—Can creep.

Eleven months—Can walk if led by one hand.

Twelve months—Can pull up and stand with help of furniture.

The American Academy of Pediatrics

Here are the things to watch for as listed by the American Academy of Pediatrics. Slightly different, these guidelines to development are those generally used by pediatricians in practice and are based on the Denver Developmental Screening Test. The age for each landmark is the approximate age at which 90 percent of children have accomplished that step.

One month—Eyes follow to midline. Baby regards face. While prone, lifts head off table.

Two months—Vocalizes. Smiles responsively.

Three months—Holds head and chest up to make ninety-degree angle with table. Laughs.

Four months—Holds head erect and steady when held in sitting position. Squeals. Grasps rattle. Eyes follow object for one hundred eighty degrees.

Five months—Smiles spontaneously. Rolls from back to stomach or vice versa. Reaches for object on table.

Six months—No head lag if baby is pulled to sitting position by hands.

Eight months—Sits alone for five seconds after support is released. Bears weight momentarily if held with feet on table. Looks after fallen object. Transfers block from one hand to the other. Feeds self cracker.

Ten months—Pulls self to standing position. Stands holding on to solid object (not human). Pincer grasp—picks up small object using any part of thumb and fingers in opposition. Says Da-da or Ma-ma. Resists toy being pulled away from it. Plays "peek-a-boo." Makes attempt to get toy just out of reach. Initial anxiety toward strangers.

Twelve months—Cruises—walks around holding on to furniture. Stands alone two to three seconds if outside support is removed. Bangs together two blocks held one in each hand. Initiates vocalization heard within preceding minute. Plays pat-a-cake.

Another growth scale.

How a baby discovers its body is another marker of development. Research by Dr. Harvey Kravitz, a pediatrician at Northwestern University, shows that hand activity begins within minutes after birth. Before his first day is over, every normal child studied had found and sucked some part of its hand. Other discovery points in Kravitz's scale of development are these:

hand-to-eye play	2 to 9 weeks
hand-to-head play	2 to 13 weeks
hand-to-nose play	2 to 17 weeks
hand-to-hand play	4 to 16 weeks
hand-to-foot play	11 to 27 weeks
hand-to-penis play	14 to 39 weeks
hand-to-buttocks play	24 to 38 weeks
hand-to-vagina play	28 to 50 weeks

If at any time your child seems to be falling seriously behind in any of these development stages, discuss it with your baby's doctor.

How much does a baby really know of what's going on?

A newborn baby can both taste and smell. And the sensations it gets through its skin seem to be especially strong. It enjoys being touched and patted gently, and likes the feeling of being closely wrapped. It is sensitive to heat and cold.

Babies can see, more than we realized at first. Not only do infants follow objects with their eyes as early as eighteen hours after birth, but during the first few weeks of life they can discriminate between various geometric shapes. And studies show they like to look at face patterns more than anything else.

Dr. Jerome Bruner, psychologist at Harvard, describes a one-month-old infant watching a bright red ball as it appears in his field of vision, goes behind a screen, then comes out the other side a black cube.

"Bang went the baby's heartbeat—at one month of age!" says Bruner. When the heartbeat drops, this is a measure of attention; it shows the baby is attending to something.

"Children are able to discriminate among more things in the first months of life than we ever dreamed of," says Bruner. "They can distinguish halftones of color, diagonals. On the day of birth, they can track a triangle with their eyes. By the time they are one month old, they can spot the identity of objects and know when something has been changed."

Infants are also aware of voices and often stop crying when someone talks to them.

The baby's emotional hunger.

Your baby has as much need for love and emotional fulfillment as it does for food. Without it, the baby will not develop properly. It needs to be rocked, held, carried, caressed, talked to, given all the tiny bits of tender loving care that give him something to respond to.

Several decades ago thousands of infants were dying of a condition called marasmus, a Greek word for "wasting away." It was responsible for half the deaths of babies to age one. Strangely, it was found that babies in the best institutions and hospitals often had this condition, while infants in the poorest of homes, but with a loving mother, did not. The difference was loving—tender attention—not just physical changing of diapers and feeding and then being left alone.

The emotional needs of infants are so great that it is astounding to talk to so many mothers who are unaware of its existence. Make sure your child gets all the love you can give it. Whether dirty dishes are in your sink or not, it will not remember; the love you give the baby now can form the entire foundation of his life.

Making life interesting and creative.

Life should be more than sleeping and eating and lying flat on your back, even for a newborn babe.

Your baby needs human contact and warmth. In addition to your handling, playing, and talking to the baby, it also needs to be stimulated by its environment. Play music, put up mobiles and other visual stimuli. Let the baby be in on some of the action of life.

The babies in those institutions without attention spent their entire time waiting for something interesting to happen to them—and eventually gave up. To protect them from drafts and from getting their heads stuck between bars, their cribs were lined with bumpers, which acted like blinders; they could see nothing on either side of them. The ceilings were white, there was nothing to look at. Nobody talked to these infants. They had no toys. They took their nourishment alone, from bottles that were propped up for them.

With this in mind, psychologists around the country have tried various experiments to see if stimulation can accelerate intellectual development. They find that brightly colored tassels, miniature umbrellas, odd-shaped boxes, and mobiles that wiggle all make a difference.

The children with these are more advanced in development than those without the extra stimulation.

Crib bumpers made of transparent plastic so that baby can see through make a difference, too. One Harvard psychologist, Dr. Burton White, said, "Almost at once, the infants began to rear up their heads like elephants to see what was going on."

And at two and a half months, he said, they pawed at the mobiles and tried to make them wiggle. "Apparently, they were terribly pleased by the whole business. They smiled at objects, vocalized, chuckled away in a manner no other institutionalized child in the hospital did—you could hear these children a whole ward away!

"I think we've shown clearly that enrichment procedures can produce remarkable effects on the course of early development."

6

How to Care for the Baby Without Becoming Utterly Exhausted

Even though the baby *is* darling, and it gurgles and coos, and it's a bundle of joy, and you love it, you wish that it wouldn't cry so much and soil its diapers faster than you can change them. Simultaneously, the dirty dishes are piling up in the sink, and your older child doesn't have clean underwear for school this morning, your husband is out of socks, and the beds aren't made. Suddenly it's time to fix dinner, and now the baby is crying again for *its* dinner.

By the time your husband comes home and you sit down to the dinner table, you are tired to the point of tears and you don't know whether to contain those tears that are welling up behind your tired eyes, or to cry, or to lay your head on your dinner plate and just fall asleep.

You wonder what happened to all those dreams of the joy of motherhood.

Don't despair. It will get better. And meanwhile there are a number of things you can do in those first weeks at home to increase your chances of survival and let you emerge as a whole person again.

The seven-point program on how to cope without losing your strength and sanity.

Let's face it, you *are* going to become tired, but it isn't necessary to become *totally* exhausted. Instead, if you carry out the following program, you will have enough of yourself left to really enjoy your baby and your new state of motherhood.

Here is the program. Read it, and *do* it.

1. Rest. This is the cardinal rule for all new mothers. The only way you can renew your strength, so that you can take care of your baby and still keep yourself together, is to obtain a luxurious amount of rest. Go to bed early. Take *two* naps a day for the first two weeks. Use the times when your baby sleeps to get rest for yourself. And take a nap every afternoon for at least the next two weeks. In fact, a nap in the afternoon isn't a bad idea for the next twenty-five years. Many people regularly take quick naps and find it improves their stamina tremendously.

2. Get help. This is your time to do nothing but care for your baby and yourself. And once you have the help, let them take charge and do the household chores. Don't follow them around checking the quality of their work. Find something completely different to do: fix the formula, wash your hair, read a book, or go back to sleep.

3. Let your husband pitch in. That big, strong, handsome man you married is big and strong enough to pick up a little pan and boil his own water for coffee in the morning and to fold his own socks and underwear for a few weeks. (In fact, there is no reason why he shouldn't do these chores all the time.) Let him take care of you and pamper you. He loves to be protective when you really feel weak and overburdened. Just ask lovingly and without complaining or demanding, and chances are he will be happy to be needed and part of the show.

4. Take quick breaks. Often sitting down for five or ten minutes with your feet up can make a great difference in keeping you from becoming overtired. There are a lot of minutes you can preserve for yourself, particularly if you define the time as a break.

5. Organize time. Make a list in the evening of what you want to accomplish during the next day. Underline or star items that are most important and tackle these priority jobs first. Scratch them off as you get them done. Study ways to make every task more efficient, from folding diapers to stacking dishes. And decide in advance what can be delegated to others. Organize your housework as though you were running a business and profits depended on time taken for each job. Minutes saved here and there can give you extra time to enjoy and to savor your baby. This is far better than being so busy doing things that fun becomes elusive and fleeting. You must have a block of time to use for *yourself.*

6. Don't be a perfectionist. We were always raised on the dictum "If a thing is worth doing, it is worth doing right." In general, we agree. But there are times when it is better to relax your standards. Undifferentiated perfectionism is a waste of time—you don't need to iron the sheets and the underwear or the terrycloth towels. You don't have to dry each dish—let it drain dry. (Studies show there are actually less bacteria in drain-dried dishes anyway.)

7. Let it go till tomorrow. Blasphemy? Not really. This is a special time. A time you need to get yourself back together. A time for definition and turning inward. As long as the baby has a few spare diapers left and milk for the next two meals, nothing else needs to be done. Relax. You can catch up on cleaning and washing tomorrow or next week or next month.

Shouldn't I feel guilty about not getting more done?

The more you take care of yourself now, the better you will be later. The less work you do now, the more work you can do later. Because you'll feel *good* then.

What are the essentials my baby really needs?

It needs enough food, enough warmth, dry clothes, stimulation of sights and sounds, and touch—and love. Concentrate on providing these.

Are there shortcuts I can take?

Certainly. And taking them doesn't make you less of a mother. What it really does is to free you of unnecessary chores so that you have more time for loving and cuddling and enjoying each other.

Don't bother heating the milk.

Most mothers overheat the baby's milk, often causing colic. And a ravenously hungry baby couldn't care less whether its milk is warm or cold.

Shirley discovered this quite by accident with her second boy, Bob. He was born by cesarean section after a long labor. One week out of the hospital, the moving men arrived to transport them to a half-remodeled old house with no kitchen sink and the kitchen stove balanced precariously on wooden boxes, waiting for overdue workmen.

Baby Bob, having weighed almost ten pounds at birth, and with shoulders like a football player, was in much better shape than Shirley, whose shaky knees made her less stable than the kitchen stove. With no way to heat the bottle, she took it from the refrigerator, stuck it in Bob's mouth, and felt guilty. Baby Bob made a funny expression, hesitated, tasted it again, and polished off the bottle with dispatch. He slept for the entire afternoon. She never heated a bottle again, but she frequently felt guilty.

Unnecessary guilt feelings, it turns out. Because later she ran across a scientific report that showed that it is unnecessary to heat baby milk.

If using ice cold milk bothers you, take the bottle out of the refrigerator for a few minutes before feeding time to allow it to approach room temperature.

Don't worry about protecting your baby from noise and activity.

In Africa, newborn babies are carried around on their mother's hips from as early as twenty-four hours after delivery. They are in the midst of all normal activity and receive constant tactile and social stimulation. With American babies, the emphasis is usually on quieting and protecting them. Many scientists believe the early exposure to stimulation is the reason why African babies, although usually smaller at birth, by the tenth day of life appear to be more attentive than their American counterparts. From then on during the first year of life, the African babies are usually more advanced in development.

What should I do about diaper rash?

Diaper rash is the name for the red, irritated skin of the baby's bottom that results from the irritating effects of ammonia. Sometimes there is a secondary invasion by fungus.

The urine contains a substance called urea, which gives it the characteristic odor. The normal bacteria on the baby's skin convert the urea to ammonia, and the rash results.

To prevent diaper rash, change diapers frequently. Place them loosely so that air can circulate and any ammonia that is formed will evaporate away. When you are treating diaper rash, it is frequently very helpful to leave the baby exposed so that the skin will stay as dry as possible.

Soak reusable diapers in commercial preparations designed to kill bacteria, so that the urea of the urine will not be converted to ammonia. Or better still, use disposable diapers.

Powder the baby's bottom each time the diaper is changed. Ordinary corn starch, which can be sprinkled from the sort of container from which sugar is sprinkled, makes an inexpensive but effective drying powder.

Does the umbilical cord require special care?

The umbilical cord dries and usually falls off by the time you leave the hospital. If it is still attached when you leave, you can accelerate the drying process by wiping its attachment to the skin with alcohol twice a day.

What if my baby is circumcised?

Until the penis is healed, you can prevent the glans from sticking to the diaper by applying vaseline at each diaper change. The remaining ring of foreskin should be pushed back at each diaper change until healing is complete. This usually occurs in two or three days after the circumcision.

And if my baby is not circumcised?

The foreskin should be pushed back at each diaper change until you are certain that it is sufficiently loose to retract readily.

What is colic?

Colic is an intestinal pain that some babies suffer during the first few months of life. The equivalent in adults is probably gas cramps, which sometimes occur with a virus or in response to certain foods.

In the baby it is probably due to an excessive buildup of gas causing distension of the intestines and resulting spasms of the intestinal muscles as they try to move the gas along.

In some babies it is also due to a form of allergy in which the milk irritates the intestines directly.

What can I do about colic?

Try to prevent excessive buildup of intestinal gas by burping the baby several times during the course of each feeding. Try to feed smaller amounts more often so that the natural fermentation gases of digestion will be of smaller volume.

If the baby is not breast-fed, try changing the formula because of the possibility that the colic is a form of allergy. And if you are breast-feeding, try to analyze your diet to determine if the colic is related to anything you eat that you are secreting in the breast milk.

Your pediatrician can prescribe an antispasmodic drug to give the baby to try to relax the spastic intestinal muscles that cause the pain.

Colic has been found not to occur among the Navajo Indians. They keep their babies on a papoose board, which is attached to the mother's back as she goes about her daily chores. The baby is tightly and securely bound to the board and is fed in a vertical position while attached to the board. At night the papoose board is hung on a peg, with the baby still attached, so that it sleeps in a vertical position.

The Navajo practice of keeping the baby vertical all the time, including feedings, encourages burping as a means of getting rid of excessive gas, since the gas bubbles rise. Having the baby tightly bound to the board across its abdomen keeps the abdomen from filling excessively with either food or gas. The constant movement of the baby in the vertical position attached to the mother's back as she goes about encourages the gas bubble to rise in the stomach and not to pass into the intestine.

You can apply these lessons to your colicky baby. Raise the head of the crib by tilting the mattress up, keep the baby tightly swaddled, and walk the baby about frequently. In fact, why not make a papoose board and strap the baby to it with a wide bandage across its abdomen? If you don't mind hugging a board, you'll certainly enjoy the quiet that replaces the crying of the colicky baby.

What to do to relieve the pain when your baby is in the throes of a colic attack? Try to burp him one more time. Place him across your knees and gently rub his back. Put him on his stomach on top of a hot water bottle or heating pad wrapped in a towel to keep it from being too hot against his skin.

If your baby is colicky, it's twice as important for you to get some rest and change for yourself so that you don't become tense in reaction to the baby. Your tenseness may make the baby more tense, setting up a cycle.

Colic usually ends by three months of age; even the worst and longest lasting cases are over by four months.

How to tell if your baby is allergic to milk.

You should be particularly alert to the possibility of milk allergy if you or someone else in your family has a history of it. They may say they never did like milk, or milk never agreed with them, or they may get diarrhea after drinking milk. Also be extra alert if your baby has eczema, because babies given bottle milk have eight times more eczema than babies given breast milk, and eczema rash is an allergic reaction.

Usually if a baby is allergic to milk, it will refuse to nurse from the bottle; typically the baby comes hungry to the bottle, grasps the nipple eagerly, takes a suck or two, then turns away with distaste. Or it may gulp irregularly with much thrashing about. With urging, the baby may take an ounce or two, but then spits up or vomits. If it finishes the bottle, he often has pain, gas, and frequent diarrhea.

The best way to avoid milk allergy is to give your baby breast milk. The next best thing is to try boiling the milk. This sometimes breaks down the protein in the milk sufficiently to prevent the allergic reaction. Let it cool completely, of course. Also try using evaporated milk or powdered milk. If the baby still reacts, try one of the milk substitutes such as Mullsoy, Sobee, Nutramigen, or Isomil. Keep the baby on evaporated milk diluted with water for as long as possible, even past age two if you can. Even if a child is not allergic to milk, it should not be rushed into changing from evaporated milk to whole milk.

Don't worry if your baby sucks his thumb.

Most babies suck their thumbs, some more than others. Let the baby have the bottle, breast, or pacifier as much as it wants to satisfy its sucking instinct. But if it wants to suck its thumb too, or chew its fist a bit or even a toe, it won't hurt anything.

A survey of twenty-six hundred children was made by Drs. Alfred S. and Howard S. Traisman, Chicago pediatricians. They found half of the children studied sucked their thumbs or fingers. It occurred equally in both boys and girls. Breast or bottle, feeding on schedule or by demand, or any other parameters measured seemed not to have any influence on the frequency of thumb-sucking one way or another. They found that if children are going to be thumb-suckers, with 75 percent of the children the habit begins before three months of age. The other 25 percent begin before they are a year old. Most were still at it at age two. The average age for stopping was between age three and a half and four.

Don't try to stop thumb- or finger-sucking. It represents a basic need of the child that should not to be discouraged in any way. This oral phase of personality development varies from child to child.

Don't give baby a bath every day.

Babies don't really get that dirty. Washing its bottom when you change its diapers is very important to prevent serious diaper rash. Wipe the baby's hands and face regularly also. To give the baby a total bath and hairwash twice a week is sufficient. In the summertime when the days are hot and sticky, more frequent baths are necessary to keep it cool and refreshed.

Keep baby's fingernails trimmed short.

Babies have a disconcerting habit of scratching themselves with their fingernails. Keep nails trimmed. Do it while baby is asleep. If the scratches are still a problem, put socks over the hands for naps or get the type of nightgown with a cuff that folds over the hands.

Don't sterilize the formula.

Modern formulas are prepackaged and are sterile-packed. Most pediatricians allow the babies to go on to whole milk by the third month.

Don't hand rinse diapers.

Buy a sturdy diaper pail and wash diapers every day or two so the smell doesn't become too strong. Your only problem is when the baby has a bowel movement. If you know your baby has a bowel movement at certain times—say, after it nurses—put diaper liners in the diaper at that time or use disposable diapers and simply throw them out. For the times you misjudge, if you fold the diaper inside out and hold the soiled area on the surface of the water in the toilet and flush it, you can rinse most of it away and not have to hand rinse.

Buy two-piece, terry cloth outfits.

When babies wear nightgowns and get wet, because of capillary action they get wet right up to the neck. With a two-piece outfit you only have to change the bottom, and you don't have to deal with those rubbery arms and elbows at every change.

With terry cloth, of course, or other machine-washable, machine-dryable, nonwrinkling fabric, ironing is unnessary.

Consider a diaper service or disposable diapers.

Check the economics of a diaper service or disposable diapers against the cost of regular diapers plus soap and water at home. The difference may be smaller than you think, and the convenience is nice, especially in the first few months.

What can I do if my baby is crying because it is teething?

Use a teething ring made of hard rubber or plastic. Cool it or a pacifier in the refrigerator before giving it to your baby. Rub a little bourbon or paregoric gently on the baby's swollen gums. Paregoric is a local anesthetic that your pediatrician can prescribe.

Babies often run a slight fever and have a runny nose at this time also, and this is nothing to worry about.

If you use a pacifier to help ease teething pain, use a pacifier with a guard that prevents the baby from sucking in the whole nipple. You can keep the pacifier handy by attaching a ribbon to it and pinning the ribbon to the baby's sleeve or shirt. Don't use a cord to hold the pacifier around the baby's neck, since it can become dangerously tight.

When should I start feeding solid foods, and what kind?

There are many varying opinions concerning when to advance the baby's diet. You should follow the pediatrician's recommendations. The breast-fed baby who is gaining weight at the proper rate can be kept on breast milk alone for as many as six months. But it seems to make sense that the baby will enjoy new tastes and flavors. They certainly smack their lips when they taste something that they like.

Use baby car beds so you don't have to hold the baby in the car.

This is more relaxing for you and a lot safer for your baby. The right-hand front seat is the most dangerous seat in a crash, and a sudden stop can throw the baby into the dashboard if you are simply holding him on your lap.

Use a sturdy car bed in the back seat that is anchored in some way and will not pitch forward in a sudden stop. Or you can get a car bed with a strap that holds the baby to the car bed, then use the seat belt to hold the car bed to the car seat. You can check various consumer publications at your public library for the makes of car bed that are considered the safest.

Never put a lap belt jointly around you and your baby together. Impact under such conditions would injure the baby severely.

Use a playpen.

Right from the beginning, put your baby into a playpen for some time of the day so that he becomes used to it. If you start using a playpen *after* baby learns to crawl, it will seem like a jail to it. If you start early, it will be a more acceptable routine. A child should not be left in a playpen for long intervals, but brief stays can be helpful to you when you need to be active and cannot watch him. One great time to make the playpen a habit is when you're cooking dinner. It saves worn nerves, cut fingers, and spilled food, and can be a time of fun as well as enable you to get things together peacefully for the return of your husband. Talk to Gurgling Gertie in the playpen as you move around, or when she is a few months older and more into the creative cooking thing, slip her a pan and a lid to bang around.

Get the fold-up playpen with string walls. They are handier and safer.

A schedule.

One way to organize your time is to set up a schedule for each day. Since babies and telephones and visitors and older children are unpredictable, you won't always be able to stick to it, but it will give you something to work around.

However, after a few weeks, the baby's eating habits will be fairly predictable, even if you are using demand feeding. You will have to plan your day around the feeding times.

Taking your baby in for checkups.

The one place where you absolutely do not want to take shortcuts is in your baby's checkup visits to the doctor. His health is vital, and it is your responsibility as a parent to see that he obtains the best start in life that you and medical science can give him.

Your baby should receive a physical examination every month beginning at one month and through six months. Take the baby to a private physician or a well-baby clinic as close to your home as you can find. After six months, most pediatricians feel that a checkup every three months is sufficient. It helps if your husband can accompany you so that after the baby has been checked your husband can attend to him, and you can talk undisturbed with the pediatrician.

The pediatrician will outline the immunization schedule that will protect your baby from most serious diseases. Don't put these dates off. Immunizations—essential to protect your child from serious diseases—should begin at eight weeks.

The two most important things you must not cut short.

Love. And attention. Your baby needs them most of all. And the major reason for wanting to eliminate as many frills of baby care as possible is so you will have the time and repose to give your baby all the love and attention you can. Both you and the baby will benefit from it.

Remember the studies of infants in institutions. Babies who are not held and cuddled do not develop as well as babies that are hugged and handled. The weight gain is less, and socialization and response to external stimuli are retarded.

Take time to hold your baby, give it the tender loving care of feeding, dressing, rocking, bathing, and carrying the baby about. It loves the secure feeling of something held firmly about it, so this is not the time to toss the baby about, but to give it firm support. This is why a small, enclosed space is better than a large, open crib for his first few weeks of sleeping also.

The baby loves skin-to-skin contact. And the sound of voices. Sing to it, talk to it. It doesn't matter that the baby does not know what you're saying.

The baby needs social contact. Put its bassinet or playpen in the kitchen while you fix dinner or near you when you do the housework or iron. Put a mobile near the baby's bed to look at. Touch it, cuddle it. Get a papoose carrier, front or back style, to carry baby with you later on your jaunts about town. Let the baby be around other people.

In your first few weeks at home, your only important responsibility to the baby is to feed it and to love it. Nothing else really matters. Drop all other jobs whenever you feel tired. Skip the bath, don't clean the house, have sandwiches for supper if need be, but save and cherish your time for hugging and holding and relaxing with the baby.

7

Handling Your
Relationships with
Husband,
Family, and Friends

Bringing home a baby as part of the family can intensify all
the feelings of people, enlarging them and concentrating
them and focusing them like nothing had before. Other people's reactions to you, your husband, and the baby show
amazingly clear patterns that you may not have even been
aware of before—both good and bad patterns—of helpful-
ness and warmth toward you and your husband, and also of
hostility and jealousy and pettiness.

How you act toward people in the weeks ahead and how
you guide the interactions that occur can determine how you

and your husband will stand together as a unit in the future in your relationships with other people.

You and your husband.

One would expect that coming home with a new baby would be a high point in a marriage, and yet many women reported to us that when the baby was born, it didn't bring them closer to their husbands, but actually imposed strains on the marriage and drove them apart.

Reactions varied tremendously. In most cases having a baby did bring the couple closer. Susan H. said she and her husband, Tom, both felt their relationship was better than ever after the baby was born. "I used to baby my husband a little and that stopped to a degree, and he had to adjust to it. But other than that we had no major adjustments to make."

Sally felt the same way. "Jim is mad about the baby. He rushes home to play with the baby every night."

Mary said she and Bob had adjustments to make because the baby basically took over the house and the time schedule, but these problems were minor. "It's a change, of course," she said, "But it's a fantastic experience, unbelievable. I was so thrilled, and Bob said he felt the same way."

Other relationships did not fare so well.

Danielle said, "I think I was a little standoffish toward my husband after the baby. I concentrated so much on the baby that I didn't pay much attention to him, whether consciously or unconsciously. After the second baby, everything was fine. I wasn't so uptight then."

Abigail said her feelings toward her husband changed drastically. "I was coming down hard on him for being irresponsible. I had an overwhelming feeling that everything had to be in its place, and if anything was out of order I got very tense about it.

"Once I recognized why I was getting so upset, it was better. It was my fault. I felt confronted, totally alone. My husband was being normal. He is actually a much better adjusted person than I am."

Abigail also reported that what upset her and her husband the most was interference with their cocktail hour. "Don would come home and I would want to talk to him and we never had the time. At other times when the baby needed attention, I would get angry with Don because I could feel him pressuring me just by his being there. I guess I just didn't realize how much time a baby takes."

Karen reported a similar problem. "I was used to being very much alone with Tom, very free, and all of a sudden we weren't alone anymore. He'd come home, and I'd want to sit down in the living room like we used to and have a drink and just talk, but in the back of my mind I was thinking that I'd better listen for the baby. After the first week that ended. I made it end, because I knew if I wanted to be alone with my husband I couldn't think about the baby so much. I had to put her away for a while."

Rita's situation was probably the most typical. "I felt a lot closer to my husband after the baby because we'd been through this together. It deepened our relationship a lot. But it was also more strained because we had less time for each other. There was more fighting, in fact, more disagreements in the weeks after Johnny was born than in the first five years of our marriage put together. Everything's all right now, but for the first three months it was rough."

What are the reasons for these different reactions?

Some psychiatrists say it may be as complex as the real reasons that you got pregnant. Perhaps in getting pregnant you were trying to prove something. Perhaps your relationship with your husband was not that good to begin with and you were trying to improve things by having a baby. Perhaps you tried to save your relationship and your marriage by having a child.

However, such reactions can also be caused by something as simple as the baby itself—a third person, a stranger—coming between you. Or it may be that the baby uses up all of your free time or all of your strength, so that fatigue makes you more irritable and creates tension over trivial things that both of you used to overlook.

You need to stand back and analyze your own individual situation and relationship.

What can we do to keep our relationship from changing?

Your relationship is bound to change somewhat. You have a major new factor that drastically changes your life. Now there are three of you, and so the presence of a child will by necessity change things that involved just the two of you.

The important thing is to see to it that the changes in your relationship become positive ones, enhancing the relationship even more, rather than causing it to deteriorate. You must pursue a positive program to ensure good feelings between you.

The cardinal rule to follow is for you and your husband to sit down and talk about these things. If you're not used to saying more than "How did it go at the office today?" then this can be a magnificent opportunity to open new avenues of communication between the two of you.

If you are both bashful about getting started, actually make out an agenda of things to talk about, with each of you making a separate list and then combining them. Include such things as hidden feelings you both have but have not talked about, whether you feel the other has been irritable or tense, what you can each specifically do to ease tensions for the other. And include positive things such as what you wish your philosophies to be in raising your child. You probably won't stick to the agenda after the first five minutes, but it's a great way to steer a conversation to the vital things you really should discuss.

Rule two: be more understanding. If each of you can make more allowance for short tempers and fatigue, you will note a big difference. If your husband comes upon you bathing the baby and says, "My God, you're always giving the kid a bath, he can't possibly get that dirty," don't hurl something back. Instead try something like "I know, I always seem elbow deep in the bathtub. Let me dry off the family diaper dirtier, and let's relax a bit. Why don't you fix us a drink!"

Or if you are tripping over the dog, burning the steak, and trying to quiet the baby all at the same time, your husband, instead of growling about the house always being in a mess, can call the dog, play with the baby, pat you on the rear, and tell you you're going to survive. Or he can say, "Out of here, Baby, I'm taking over."

There are ten minutes a day that are the most important of any in your relationship: the first five minutes when you greet in the morning and the first five minutes you are together when you or he comes home. What you say in those minutes sets up a positive or negative attitude, sets the tone for the day or evening.

Make sure, no matter how tired you are, no matter how discouraged you are, no matter how bad the boss or the kids have been, in those first five minutes you both treat each other with love and tender understanding. Then it will follow, with the ambiance established, that the following hours will be more pleasant.

Shall the baby sleep in your room?

It's best for a baby to have its own room. If you must have the baby in your room now, limit its stay. Find another room for it within a month or so. You may be disturbed by the baby and he may be disturbed by you.

And don't worry about being with your baby every minute listening to its breathing. A new baby's breathing is irregular. If you are lying awake in the night listening to its breathing, you will hear it sigh, hold its breath, and pant. None of this is reason to get upset.

If you have your bedroom door open you can hear if the baby cries.

Going out.

Go. You both need it. And don't worry about the baby. It will be all right. If you come rushing home, anxious and worried, you'll find it blissfully sleeping and totally unconcerned.

Other times, take the baby with you. The new baby will probably sleep right through a square dance or a picnic just as well as a bridge game.

We don't recommend long or difficult travel at first, however. Neither mother nor baby are up to long trips. Postpone them awhile. And it's best that you two don't go off on a vacation leaving the baby at home with others right after it is born. The baby needs that first loving contact and recognition during the early months of life.

Postpartum depression in men.

You may have heard of husbands having symptoms of pregnancy along with their wives. It is more common than generally realized. In fact, Dr. Jack Valpey, obstetrician–gynecologist with a U.S. Army Hospital in Germany, interviewed three hundred couples and found at least 20 percent of men said they had symptoms during their wives' pregnancies and even took time off from work and saw doctors.

Some husbands also have sympathetic suffering during the postpartum period, experiencing some of the same symptoms as their wives. It is not uncommon for husbands to be hospitalized during the postpartum period with attacks of abdominal pain, or even appendicitis. This represents a psychophysiological reaction, indicating that both psychological and physical stresses are felt by husbands at this time.

Jealousy and what to do about it.

"And baby makes three" is not always a good feeling. It was your domain and now you suddenly have to share it with your baby.

With Frieda the jealousy was even more direct. "I suddenly felt I had to compete with the baby for my husband's attentions. That was a new feeling and I didn't like it. When he steps in the door, what's he going to do—embrace me or kiss the baby?"

The husband feels jealousy too. He wonders if his wife and baby are joined in some kind of unholy alliance. They're always with each other and at each other and part of each other. Where is there room for him?

Sara said she didn't believe her husband when he said, "If it's a boy, I might be jealous." Then, she said, "Astoundingly, I found he was!"

More husbands than you might think display tremendous jealousy after the child's birth, sometimes outwardly, sometimes in more hidden ways—such as tension and irritability

—which you might not think are caused by jealousy.

Chances are the jealousies that both of you feel are embarrassing to you. But you'll find tremendous relief if you can bring them to the surface and discuss them.

More serious problems.

Sometimes problems arise in this period that cannot be overcome by simply discussing them. Sometimes the marriage really isn't solid. And the couple has thought that having a baby would resolve their problems. Usually this just doesn't work.

Kaye reported: "It was very strange. He started drinking, heavily. Our whole relationship became different. Anybody can take a drink. The problem is that he gets wild. He even gets upset and frustrated if I get tired. We can either resolve it or separate."

Husbands must know where they belong in the family picture, or the new baby can bring on not a strengthening of the marriage, but a breakdown.

When problems become as serious as this, you should seek professional help. Call your obstetrician first and consult with him. He may want to talk to both you and your husband in his office to try to help you. Or he may refer you to a marriage counselor, psychologist, or psychiatrist to help you probe deeper into the factors troubling your relationship.

If your husband doesn't seem to love the baby.

Give him time. He may be jealous or he may feel left out or ignored. Show him in as many ways as you can that he is still loved and needed—by you and the baby. Encourage him to help in feeding and bathing the baby, but if he seems reluctant, don't force it.

He will eventually get used to the new member of the family. As one young mother said, "Why shouldn't my husband feel strange with the baby? They just met each other a couple of weeks ago!"

Try feeding the baby while sitting and talking with your husband, so he will feel part of the picture. Talk about the baby together. Discuss present problems and future decisions: What are the characteristics you want to encourage in your child most? What are some of the things you want to do together? Do you want other children? How many? How soon? What are the family histories on both sides? What family traits do you want to encourage or discourage? Talk about the mystery of what your baby will grow up to be like and the ways you can love it and guard it and support it and help prepare it for independence and meeting the world on its own. For parents must play a dual role—holding close the child in love and sending it away, out into the world.

As you discuss all these things about the baby, you'll be surprised what you learn about yourselves also.

Special things the husband can do.

"There are times when my husband leaves a mess, leaves a real trail behind him. The first week I was home he came in drunk. He was rebelling, and also in a way he was so worried about the baby being normal. That's why he didn't bring a camera into the delivery room, he didn't have enough faith that everything would be okay."

That was Cynthia, depressed because of the lack of support she received from her husband during the trying postpartum period.

Many women we talked to said they had an overwhelming feeling of being alone after the baby was born. Probably the most important single thing a man can do at this time is to give his wife emotional support. Show her you are part of what is happening and are happy about it. Show her that you love her and the baby, that you feel close and intimate.

Try not to feel neglected during the time she spends with the baby. But if you do feel neglected and jealous, talk about it in a nonaggressive way so you can work it out and even laugh about it together.

And don't get angry or upset if your wife gets depressed and goes on crying jags. She hates it as much as you, can't help it, and needs your support more than ever.

Get to know your baby, really know it. Let yourself be uninhibited and loving, even if you feel awkward at first. There's nothing unmanly about being tender. Pick the baby up, hold it, closely and warmly. Just avoid sudden, jerking movements. Don't hold it at arms' length, but lovingly against your chest. Feel its fuzzy head and little round bottom. Talk to it about all the great things you want it to know about life. Hold the baby against your bare chest. The skin-to-skin contact makes the baby feel secure and the father feel good.

Pitch in and help your wife. She'll love help with the dinner and laundry. But don't limit it to the nonbaby things. If you can run an office or fix a car motor, you can also make it through the intricacies of warming a bottle, changing a diaper, or giving the baby a bath. It will draw you and your wife closer than you can imagine, and you will be satisfied to be really sharing in your new baby's life. And you want this baby to know you as a warm, comforting person, not just the deep voice from across the room. If you are a part of your child, it will be a strong bond drawing you to your family each night.

What the husband can do when the wife is in the hospital.

Read the books she reads and discuss the ideas presented in them.

Try to arrange for her to have a telephone to call her friends.

Try to arrange for her to have rooming-in if she wants it so she can have the baby with her.

During your visits, take some powder for a back rub.

Bring fruit if she is allowed to have snacks.

Bring her vitamins, stationery, books, or whatever she might have forgotten or needs.

Help her make arrangements with the doctor at the time to go home.

Bring the baby clothes when you come to pick her up.

Support her in breast-feeding if she wants to do this.

Love her, talk to her, be enthusiastic, and warm and tender.

What a husband can do when the baby comes home.

Help your wife plan and arrange the baby's room.

Help her find and decide on someone to help with the

housework and child care. (If she does not want your mother or hers to help, do not insist.)

Support her in doing her exercises and following her diet.

Do not demand your supper the moment you walk in from work.

Help cook or get the dinner on the table if she is busy with the baby.

Help her, but don't underestimate her. She's a woman and wants to do her job well.

Get her to go out frequently for walks and to a movie or for dinner.

Pick up after yourself and help any older child do likewise. (Why not all the time? Why should somebody have to pick up after a grown man?)

Do not push her about sex. And try forms of lovemaking other than coitus. (See Chapter 13.) Right now, lots of affection can be even more important to her than sex.

Parents and in-laws.

Feelings toward your parents can be very complex during early motherhood. They may be strengthened by the baby's coming. They may remain the same or they may be changed radically for the worse.

Ann said she had never been close to her father because he was always so busy. "But when I came home with the baby, everyone except him was away. My mother was in Europe and my in-laws were in Japan. We had a whole relationship with the baby that was really lovely, and then had a continuing relationship after that which hadn't existed before."

Other new mothers say that their parents and their in-laws drive them up the wall because they try to tell them how to take care of the new baby. "My mother has always treated me like a child," Sandy said. "I thought when I became a mother of a ten-pound boy, she would begin treating me like an adult. But no, now she treats us all like children: me, my six-foot three-inch, forty-year-old, vice-president husband, and the new baby."

What you can do to improve relations in the generation gap.

One thing you can do is try to keep from setting up defenses. Don't bristle before your mother or mother-in-law even arrives on the scene. And don't automatically reject the suggestions made by mothers. Keep an open mind and think about the suggestions with the same objectivity that you give to suggestions from a friend. Some of the suggestions might just be good ones!

If your mother or mother-in-law on the other hand really nags, attacks, and criticizes, don't accept the hostility and criticism blindly. Try with your answers to work toward establishing the point that you have your own ideas and your own life to lead. Try to stand up for your own rights without being hostile or aggressive.

Games to recognize.

Learn to recognize the games being played and the roles being acted out among your relatives.

Ann found her husband and his mother teaming up almost like parents and treating her like a child. "Richard and I don't think Ann should continue her sculpture studio now. It's just too much for her."

Or you may find your mother setting up a flirtation with your husband and competing with you in conversation and in other ways, reminding you perhaps of similar situations when you were younger, when your mother overcharmed your male callers and made you feel like a dud.

It's not always easy to recognize games in action, and being the young, new mother, you may feel too young and unsure of yourself or even too respectful to do anything about such a situation. But once you see a repeating pattern of behavior that is disrupting to your relationship with your husband, you should try to be strong enough to talk it over with him and do something together to head off trouble.

Even if you can't change your in-laws and their long-established behavior patterns, at least you and your husband can have a united front. You can accept the fact that there is a problem without blaming each other, you can support each other against attack rather than blindly standing up for your parents against your husband, you can talk over ways to try to diminish the problem or avoid it.

In analyzing a given situation you must first determine who is doing what to whom. And why. Is the mother who reared such a terrific man as your husband really such a bitch? Or are you overreacting, so unsure of yourself you can't consider suggestions on their own merits?

What effect is the game having? A running battle of trivia, or is a mother-in-law successfully dividing and conquering you and your husband, constantly driving you apart? Is she domineering and still ordering her son around? Or are you so overly possessive that you are not permitting her to continue love and reasonable companionship with her son?

Once you have analyzed the situation, then you can take steps to build a happy, positive relationship, instead of the destructive one now in effect. How much happier and more rewarding for everyone!

You and your mother.

Whatever your relationship with your mother, now that you have a baby, it will be intensified. If your relationship is good, it will now be enhanced. If it was none too good before, all hell may break loose now. You'll fight your old battles over the new child.

If you are typical, you probably secretly hope that you will do a better job of raising your child than your mother did with you. In fact, if typical, you probably wish deep down that she will also tell you that you are doing a superior job.

In turn, she, if typical, feels if you raise your child differently from the way she did, you are really criticizing her methods.

So you're both uptight. You wonder if you're doing as good a job as your mother did. And she wonders why you think her way was wrong.

Actually, you both had the same goal in mind—to raise your child to the best of your ability and in line with your own convictions. She made some mistakes, and if you are human, you will make some too.

Try to profit from her mistakes without being uptight about them. If your relationship was so bad that you simply can't forget the past and can't solve the present, then at least don't feel guilty about it.

Some answers.

The answers are not easy.

They basically involve self-strength. Your husband and you must be a unit, must have strength between you to share your new responsibilities and still retain your warmth and closeness and special feeling for each other.

With this as a basis, you can formulate together what your policies will be toward other people, whether they be relatives, friends, or others outside your family. Many of the problems of these interrelationships that seemed insurmountable when faced alone become relatively manageable when the two of you sit down and discuss them and map out a plan with which to attack them.

Knowing that these problems are apt to occur, forewarned as you now are, you can be alert for the signs of difficulties and can do much to prevent them. Or knowing that others have come through the same problems, it can give you the strength and the humor to weather them until sun shines through again.

Most important of all will be your own strength, which you can build up and rely on. Many of the women we interviewed found this out the hard way.

As one said, "It wasn't really a problem with my friends or my mother or my husband. My problem was with myself. If someone had sat down and talked with me and told me what to expect, I think it would have helped. Anything to pull me out."

Advice to grandparents.

What we need in this country is a practical guidebook for beginning grandparents. There are many things that grandparents can do to ease the problems of the generation gap at new motherhood time.

The first thing they can do is treat the new parents as adults. It's about time. They are no longer children when they have children of their own. By removing the parent–child relationship, the parties concerned can begin to treat each other with the respect of adults and build an entirely new relationship and greater appreciation than they ever had before. Realize that any criticism you give is going to be strongly resented, so try to limit your suggestions or mix them with an equal amount of praise for how your new parents are handling their baby. Even safer is to buy a book that says the things you want to say and present that to the new parents. You might even mark things in the margins about how such and such worked so well when you had Mary as a baby. Putting things in warm terms of "you know that worked marvelously when you were a baby . . ." will be accepted a lot sooner than aggressively hinting that your daughter isn't doing right with her baby.

Other rules: Never refer to the baby as "It." Don't criticize the name they chose whether you like it or not. It's their baby, and they can name it anything they want. And if *they* choose to say "it," that's *their* privilege.

Don't use baby talk. It's not "milkee," it's milk.

Never put down modern conveniences such as disposable diapers just because you didn't have them.

Don't discourage your daughter or daughter-in-law from breast-feeding. It will be best for her and the baby. Encourage her. On the other hand, if she feels strongly that breast-feeding is not for her, don't make this an issue between you. It's *her* business.

In fact, positive encouragement is what she needs most from you in every situation. Encouragement can be the most valuable thing you as a grandparent can give the new parents.

Other things you can do: Come over with a camera you can handle well and take lots of pictures. Do the shopping. Drive your daughter places if she doesn't have a car to get around with the new baby. Offer enthusiastically to baby-sit for the new parents, to give them a chance to get out on their own again and have some freedom to renew their husband and wife bonds.

Above all, remember the classic ways of describing in-laws: nagging, critical, meddlesome, jealous, competitive, domineering, antagonistic. Think over carefully how you act toward your son's and daughter's new family and make sure none of these adjectives describe you.

How to handle visitors.

On your first day home from the hospital, no visitors. Your first day home should be for yourself. Not just because you're tired, but also because the day is special. It's the first day for the three of you alone together. It's like riding a bike for the first time: a combination of unsureness, of learning, and a giddy, euphoric feeling of "This is it!"

Enjoy it, but don't push yourself. It's a physically and emotionally exhausting day. Don't do a bit of work. Let your husband bed both you and the baby down early for a good night's sleep.

It's not a day for entertaining friends and relatives, and your husband should protect you from them. One terrific idea is to put a sign on the door. "Mother and daughter doing fine. 6 lbs. 3 oz. Name: Mary Sue. Everybody sleeping now. Please call tomorrow." A message on a tape recorder can also intercept calls. Take them when you want to be sociable. Put on the recorder when you don't, simply saying you are asleep and will return the call at a later time.

On this day or other days, it is simple for your husband, your mother, or your housekeeper to answer the phone. She can say, "Mrs. Jones is resting (or feeding the baby or whatever) now. Would you care to leave a message? She can return your call later today or tomorrow."

In most cultures, families and friends hover over the mother and new baby much more than in our present culture. In certain societies of Central America, for example, the new mother is bundled up with her baby in swaddling clothes for several weeks while she becomes adjusted to her baby. In areas of Africa, village women bring food to the household and relatives do the housework, while the new mother spends her time recovering and getting to know herself as a mother.

In Japan the new mother is kept in bed for three weeks, preferably in the hospital. All chores are performed for her except for breast-feeding and her own personal hygiene.

In our culture, a relative often comes in for a week to help with housework and the baby, but not always. Sometimes relatives live far away in our very mobile society, or often a couple has divorced itself emotionally from family and is forced to be independent. The implementation of independence can also carry a built-in burden of loneliness. If this is true in your case, it is doubly important that you and your husband be close in this period.

On the other hand, you may be besieged by friends and relatives during the entire event. In this case, accept help and gifts graciously, and with the same warmth and spirit they are given. And enjoy the company and good feelings, but don't feel obliged to entertain. If you are too tired to see anyone, be frank about it. And when company is there, don't wait on them, let them help themselves and wait on you.

Getting along with the neighbors and other new mothers.

The most important thing, especially in the beginning, is to set up the schedule that you think is best for you and your husband and your baby, and then stick to it. If a friend wants to come over and visit, and you would rather go to bed or spend the evening alone with your husband or read a book, then feel free to say that you just don't feel up to a social evening. Suggest an alternate time to assuage hurt feelings.

When it comes to advice on rearing children and caring for babies, keep an open mind. Someone, even a grandparent, just might have a good idea, and it pays to listen objectively. But if someone makes a suggestion that simply does not coincide with your and your husband's philosophy of baby care, then do not feel intimidated into accepting it. You can simply ignore the advice or state that you prefer to handle it a different way.

Be polite and friendly to your neighbors, of course. Sitting in the sun in the backyard or the park watching your babies grow up together can be good fun, and other mothers can become great friends. But if you don't want to become part of a regular coffee klatch routine, then don't let yourself get caught in the habit. If someone comes in and seems content to stay for the morning, and you are busy, then you can simply explain that you must get to the laundry or bank or someplace. Then you can leave the house together.

Don't compete with other mothers.

We knew a woman in a Chicago suburb who always had the cleanest children and cleanest house in town. Her children were always scrubbed and wore immaculate, beautifully ironed dresses, and they would go home sobbing heartbroken if they got their clothes dirty when playing in the sandbox. Her kitchen floor was scrubbed every day, her furniture was polished three times a week, and her windows were washed every ten days. On schedule. Never a thing out of place. But she was so busy keeping her house spotless that she never had time for friends. In five years she never had a party. The only people who saw the inside of her spotless house were her husband and her relatives who came to visit once a month. On schedule.

Relax. Life is not a contest. Determine your style, what is really important to you. And do it your way.

Stay out of the comparing babies game.

Whether your baby's first tooth comes in before Sally's baby's or whether he says "dada" a month sooner or later is not going to determine which of them graduates cum laude from Harvard Law School. Babies progress in different ways and at their own paces.

When dear old Sally smugly goes into her routine about her Superbaby who seems to have cut its first tooth at one week, walked at three weeks, and said supercalifragilisticexpealidocious at three months, try to think of pleasant thoughts like a seashore at misty dawn or Sally taped up in a mummy's mask unable to open her mouth for 5,000 years. When she deprecatingly asks when *your* (obviously mentally retarded) baby accomplished these great feats, smile sweetly and say that you really don't keep track of such things, but you are sure it was within the normal range of growth development as outlined by Drs. Gesell, Ginott, and Hootenanny. Then ask her the deepest philosophical question you can think of from the latest novel you've read. It should at least serve to change the topic of conversation.

If your baby sucks well, reacts to sudden noises, heeds voices, is visually alert, makes some kind of vocal sound, and smiles by around three months, relax . . . it's doing fine.

Hostile comments and how to understand them.

Many people, including members of your family, will be awed by your capabilities with your new baby. They will be threatened by the real or imagined inner knowledge that their performance in the same role was not as good as yours. This will make them feel guilty. Because this guilt is a result of your good baby management, they will feel inner resentment of you and will frequently express hostility toward you.

Carol's mother would say, "You shouldn't take the baby into an air-conditioned room." This comment projected this grandmother's feeling of hostility. Carol learned not to react personally but would answer, "My doctor says it is all right," even though the doctor was never asked.

Your doctor will always back you up in such a situation.

What should I tell visitors who have colds?

Tell them you would really love to see them but your doctor has told you not to expose yourself or your new baby to cold germs. Anyone who has a cold or has been sick in any way should know not to visit a new baby.

If you have a cold, it would even be best for you not to handle the baby. But many times this is impossible. At least wear a gauze mask, try not to breathe on the baby or cough near him, and wash your hands thoroughly before you pick the baby up.

How to present the baby to other children.

No matter how old or young your other children are, they should be made to feel part of the event of a new addition to the family. You should start out with the sharing during pregnancy. Buy a book with pictures of a growing fetus so that you can explain to your child how the new baby is developing from time to time. You can explain the various stages, such as when it has fingers and when it begins to move. This will increase your child's fascination with the whole mystery of life. Let the child feel your abdomen and the baby's movements. Explain that when the baby is ready to be born, you will go to the hospital for it to be born. This will help the child prepare for the separation when you go to the hospital. Tell your young child that you are going to the hospital so that the doctor can help you at this important time. Otherwise, a very young child may suspect that terrible things may be done to you in the hospital.

Let the child help decorate what will be the new baby's room. If he has to make a change, such as giving up a crib, stress that he is graduating to a more grown-up stage, not that he is being pushed out.

When the baby comes home, be sure to include older children in the celebration. Give them extra attention so they don't feel they are losing your love.

Let them help. Talk things over and let them know how tired you are and how much you need their help. Let them give a bottle to the baby or bring you milk and cookies in bed.

Your older child is bound to show some jealousy, but usually talking it over plus spending extra time with him will solve the problem.

But sometimes the jealousy is more serious. Mary's older son Gregory, aged two, really gave her a hard time. "For the first week he refused to speak to me," she said. "He was horrible about the baby. He didn't do anything to the baby himself, but when my husband or I held the baby, he'd jump up on the couch or jump on us. Sometimes he would throw things around or he'd hit everybody in sight."

If such behavior goes on for several weeks without improvement, you should talk to your doctor about getting some professional help.

The jealous child does not even realize he is jealous. All he knows is that he seems to be deprived of something that he previously had. He doesn't want to play second fiddle. He needs special understanding and reassurance that he is still important to you and that you love him very much.

Try not to talk about the baby all the time. Cuddle with

your older child as often as you can. Bring him an occasional present so it isn't always the new baby who is getting presents.

Other signs of jealousy.

Sometimes signs of jealousy will not be so obvious. The older child may want to act like a baby again himself. He may want to have a bottle again. Go ahead and let him. It won't hurt anything. Or he may talk baby talk or wet his bed at night or not eat well or have frequent accidents. Don't become upset, he will work it out as you give him extra love and he knows he is not displaced.

How to deal with hostility in siblings.

Hostility in the older brother or sister is natural and normal. The older sibling will feel guilty about these hostile feelings if he sees only positive feelings expressed by the parents toward the new baby.

It is therefore very good to tell the older sibling, "Sometimes I get very angry at baby Billy when he cries." This reassures the older sibling that feelings of anger are allowed and natural.

How to handle breast-feeding when there are other children.

It is all right to let the other children see you nurse the new baby since it's a natural function they should be familiar with. But seeing you and the baby in such intimacy is apt to make the older children feel their jealousy even more, so it is best at least most of the time to nurse the baby away from them.

You should repeatedly reassure the older sibling, "When you were a baby I fed you like this also. Each baby gets its turn to be fed like this." You should assert this even if you did not breast-feed the older child.

What to do if your two-year-old wants some too.

If he or she really seems to want it badly, it is best to let them try the breast milk again rather than make them feel rejected. Chances are it won't taste so good after cow's milk anyway and it will only be a one time thing.

Tell the older child who wants to try it to get a spoon and expel some of your milk into a spoon. The older child will prefer cold milk from the refrigerator.

You may also want to buy the older child a baby doll with bottles and let him feed his baby doll while you feed your baby.

Your baby and pets.

You can let your dog or cat examine the new baby. But be sure to observe the pet's reaction to the baby many times before leaving them alone together. In fact, it is better to be safe and not leave them alone at all.

You and your obstetrician.

The old tradition was that the woman fell in love with her obstetrician, worshipped him with blind trust, and did whatever he said without question. Now the picture is different. Women are learning about their bodies and they want to know the reasons for the instructions they get on what to do.

Patients are still patient, but they're no longer passive. And we think that the change in attitude is healthy.

Of course you should like your physician and trust his professional judgment and competence. If you don't like him or he's a male chauvinist, you should find another doctor.

Since you came through the last nine months with your doctor, we'll assume you like him. What's important now is that you keep in touch with him. Call him if you have any problem. Confide in him. Feel free to ask him anything. Work with him, not against him. And always be frank with him. He can't treat you competently if he doesn't have all the facts and know your feelings. If he is not meeting your needs you must tell him how he could be more effective. If he is not responsive you should consider changing.

Don't ever be timid about asking questions. If you understand why you are doing things, you will be more likely to carry out the instructions and stick to the advice.

And remember your body is yours. Final decisions about

it, such as sterilization or contraception, are yours, and not your doctor's. He can talk to you and advise you about medical complications and various factors you should be aware of, but the final decisions are yours.

Unfortunately, the legal system has not caught up with women's rights yet. Many states still require the consent of the husband before abortion or sterilization procedures can be performed on a married woman. It is not uncommon to see women with as many as fifteen children denied voluntary sterilization when they want it desperately but their husbands withhold consent. And in other states, permission for abortions or sterilization can only be given with the approval of a committee of physicians.

Don't automatically put your doctor down just because it's the current fad. Most physicians in ob–gyn have chosen that specialty because of the joy of bringing children into the world, and your doctor has a great deal of respect for the women he comes in contact with every day.

"One of the beautiful things about this job," one ob–gyn told us, "is that you are in touch every day with the marvelous miracle of birth and new life. And then you see a woman at first unsure of herself, ill at ease, grow into a mother, composed and serene, who now is in control of herself and her baby. It's a beautiful thing to see, and every time it happens, I'm happy to be part of it."

8

Getting Help Around the House

Elaine's story was a typical one.

"After I had the baby home for five weeks, I was standing in his room, and I just wanted to throw him out the window, or give him away. I didn't want to be a mother. I didn't want a child. I wanted my life back to normal. I had to get out. I got a baby-sitter and left. I cried all the way in the taxi.

"I wish that someone had told me I should go out and resume my own life a little bit. I should have been told to get someone in the house and go out two or three afternoons a week, since we can afford it, and do what I wanted. I shouldn't have been allowed to sit there and wallow. I'm going to be smart for the next one. I'm going to make all of the arrangements ahead of time for help."

Getting help is one of the most important things you can do to get back on your feet after delivery and to avoid some of the overpowering fatigue of the first few weeks. Help at home will give you the opportunity to get away from the routine of care and to deal with the emotional upsets of the postpartum period.

When should you make arrangements for help?

The help that you want for the first week or two at home should be arranged before you go to the hospital. It is also helpful, but not always possible, to line up help that you will want after that, such as a baby-sitter and a once-a-week cleaning woman.

What is the best kind of help to have?

That depends partly, of course, on your personality and your needs. But we feel the ideal person would have the following characteristics:
- unobtrusive, yet vigorous and energetic
- quiet, easy to get along with
- acknowledges mother as the person in charge
- happy to do anything necessary to help you
- comfortable with children if you have older children to take care of
- has had children herself

How to deal with whoever will help.

More important than whom you choose to help you is your ability to deal effectively with that person. You need to analyze what are your most important needs that she can fulfill, and which things you want to do yourself. There are certain jobs that you may consider fun to do yourself or that you might resent the other person doing. Once you have analyzed just how you wish to use your help, whether it be paid or volunteer help, be sure to spell out carefully what you would like to have done so the person completely understands her duties. Then step back and let that person do it without hovering.

What are the best duties for a helper?

Some new mothers like to have experienced help with the baby and so prefer a baby nurse who will help with bathing and feeding.

But in reality, the chores that center around the baby are the easiest, the least tiring, and the most important ones for you to master yourself. After all, they will finally be yours to do. It is much more sensible for you to have a helper to do all your household chores, particularly those that require the most energy.

We believe that your helper should do the laundry and cleaning, the meal preparation, and dishes. The helper can look after older brothers and sisters and run errands and shop. And you can rest and feed the baby and entertain your friends and relatives who come to admire the new baby and exchange stories of deliveries and recoveries. Or the helper can keep an eye on the baby if you want to spend some time with your older child, who may be finding the advent of the new baby difficult.

What can you expect a baby nurse to do?

A "baby nurse" may or may not be a nurse. Usually she is not a nurse, but rather is someone who has assigned that title to herself to designate her role as a helper for a new baby.

She will usually do all the baby-related chores such as bathing and diapering and feeding the new baby. She will frequently do light housekeeping, but usually expects her meals to be prepared, and she usually expects someone else to clean the house.

You must define her duties before you hire her.

One of the nice things about having her—in addition to the fact that she helps prevent you from becoming overly tired —is that having her there builds up your self-confidence.

As Jean said: "Bathing the baby was one thing that I was terrified about. The baby was slippery and wet, and I would have control with only one hand. And washing the hair! . . . I knew I couldn't wash the kid's head. I had a nurse for the first week. If I hadn't, the baby would have drowned. I was frightened at cleaning the eyes and cleaning the ears, anything that was delicate. I had no idea how to clip nails, and I cut her finger with the cuticle scissors once. I just didn't know what I was doing. Now I'm such an expert there's nothing that frightens me."

Rivalry between the baby nurse and the new mother.

"After I came home, we hired a baby nurse, to have somebody to relieve me and show me what to do." It was Nancy speaking. "But there was also a sense that she had her own system that might interfere with what I wanted to do. Like she told me I shouldn't hold the baby because I would spoil her. I told her it was my baby and I'd spoil her if I wanted to. A mother has to do what *she* thinks is right."

Frequently you will feel instinctively that your helper is doing something wrong, as in Nancy's story. You must listen to yourself first and realize that your instincts will usually be right.

This is not a time to be intimidated by the baby nurse or mother or mother-in-law. It is a time to say, "I know it should be done as I feel," as Nancy knew that she should pick up the baby when she wanted to. If you feel insecure about expressing yourself, or if you hesitate to hurt your mother-in-law's feelings by disagreeing with her, you can always say, "My doctor says that it should be done this way." You can thus depersonalize the confrontation.

It is important that the husband feel free to differ with the nurse also. Some husbands will back up the nurse automatically because they are afraid the wife really doesn't know anything about infant care, and this can be very upsetting to the inexperienced mother.

How can you find a baby nurse?

Often there are nurse registries listed in the yellow pages. You can contact your local Visiting Nurse Association, or your obstetrician may well know of someone.

Should a baby nurse be an R.N. or can she be an L.P.N.?

An R.N. is a registered nurse, which means she has probably gone to college or has taken a four-year nursing course in a hospital. She is licensed to administer medications and treatments, and it is unlikely that she will work in the home as a mother's helper.

An L.P.N. is a licensed practical nurse. She has had a shorter training period, and in most states cannot administer medications unless she is supervised by a registered nurse. An L.P.N. is paid less and will often work in the home.

Either one is satisfactory as a baby nurse if they love children and have had experience with babies.

You can have a nurse live in, come in for eight hours a day, or come in as a visiting nurse, simply stopping by to check on you and the baby and give any necessary medications or advice.

Where can I find a good cleaning woman?

First, you might ask your doctor and his nurse. They often keep lists of women who like to take new baby cases. Be sure that they know whether you want a baby nurse or someone who will mainly take care of the house.

Ask your friends if they have help who have any extra days free or who have friends who are looking for work. Be sure to check references and to interview the person before you go to the hospital. After you are home is no time to find out the person is not to your liking. In fact, it would be a good idea to have her come in to work for several days before you go to the hospital. Then your house and laundry will be in good shape before you go, she can learn her way around your house, and you can have a chance to get used to each other.

You may also want to check an employment service, which will charge a fee, or you may want to call your nearest state employment office, which will not charge a fee.

Check on the usual wages for maids in your area so you can arrive at an agreement on this in advance.

Some family service agencies may also be able to recommend a "homemaker," a reliable woman who will come in daily for a period and keep the home functioning for your husband and other children.

Live-in versus a day worker.

A live-in helper usually is on duty six days and evenings per week. She is not actually caring for the baby or doing housework the entire time, day and night, of course, but is available for any special needs, such as the nighttime feeding of the baby.

A regular live-in maid will do the heavy cleaning as well as the laundry, shopping, cooking, etc. Another type of live-in is the mother's helper or college girl who for room and board and a small salary baby-sits and also does light housekeeping, meal preparation, and dishes. Often these girls do not do heavy cleaning, however.

A day worker comes in to work only for the day, usually nine to five or nine to four. By having a day worker come in two or three days a week you can have the cleaning, laundry, and shopping pretty well taken care of, and she can prepare the evening meal before leaving. The other nights you or your husband can prepare the meals.

Interviewing prospects.

Whether you decide on a baby nurse or a housekeeper, you need to conduct an interview before you go to the hospital.

Before the person being interviewed arrives, you should decide on exactly what you want done, the hours you wish her to work, and what wages you are willing to pay. You might like to make a list of the duties you want her to perform and give her a duplicate to take home.

When you interview her, be sure to ask for the names, addresses, and telephone numbers of one or two families she has worked for recently. If she forgets them, ask her to telephone them when she returns home. And be sure to call the people and actually check them out to see if they found her satisfactory.

At the interview, the essentials to determine are whether the person is neat, has a positive attitude about the job, has a likable disposition, has a way with children, and is in good health.

Try her out in advance if at all possible. This is especially important if there are other children in your family, so that they have a chance to get used to her while you are still at home.

Should I let my mother help at first?

Your mother or mother-in-law can be the most understanding person of all to help you out if the two of you get along well. If you don't get along, it can change weeks of what should be happiness and contentment into weeks of tension and frustration.

This is one of the areas where reactions of new mothers have differed tremendously.

Rachel was glad her mother was with her. "It made a big difference. She was great about knowing everything."

Ruth said, "I didn't let my mother come until Ned was a month old, and I wish now that I had let her come right away because she has proven to be very fair. She doesn't try to tell me what to do at all, I think because *her* mother always tried to tell *her* what to do, and she knows. Pete's mother drives me crazy, but that's because she always drives me crazy. I dislike her so much I don't even want her to enjoy the baby even though I do because I have to."

Another young woman had the same kind of experience. "I would have kept my mother there forever. She stayed for two and a half weeks. I got along with her very well. As a matter of fact, she has arthritis and is a chronic complainer, but when she saw the baby, she stopped worrying about what was wrong with her, even getting up in the middle of the night to feed the baby. But Joe's mother came three days later. We don't get along at all. She finally left. My mother is coming again next month because I begged her to."

Another woman with a new baby found her feelings very defensive. "Now I finally felt on my own and I didn't want advice from my mother because I disagree with her views so much. I finally felt that I could counter the argument that she and Dad had used for many years: 'Some day you'll be a parent and then you'll understand!' "

Sometimes becoming a mother yourself will change the attitudes you have toward your own mother, transforming the entire relationship. One girl reported: "When I would say, 'The baby wants attention,' my mother would kiddingly say, 'Well, you wanted a tremendous amount of attention when you were a baby.' And I'd say, 'Gee, you never told me that before.' My relationship with her is different now."

Louise had the same type of change. "I thought I was always right and was a little smug. But after I had the baby for a few months, I started looking back at my mother, realizing I had been putting her down all these years as just being a mother. But it's some job. So of course I look at her much differently now, and our relationship has gotten much better."

You will have to make your own decision about whether your mother or mother-in-law will be a real help to you. Naturally having one of them to help out is financially cheaper than paying for a maid or nurse. You have to balance the monetary savings against the emotional expenditures involved.

How can I say NO if my mother offers to help me?

This is a good time to use your "Doctor's Orders" ploy. Rather than engage a well-meaning grandmother in a confrontation in turning down her offer of help because it may be unpleasant or because she may be a hindrance, you can easily state, "My doctor believes that this is a better time to have paid help," or something to that effect.

Do you think it's a good idea for husbands to help instead of hiring someone?

Your husband is of course going to be helping with many things. Some husbands go even further than the average and take a week or two of vacation time to be home with the new mother and baby and share or take over the work of house-cleaning and meals.

Just as you interview and instruct paid help prior to the delivery and your return home from the hospital, you must help your husband prepare himself. Starting long in advance you can make lists of chores and schedules so that he will be able to help you in an organized fashion. You can prepare menus for your first two weeks at home and even do most of the shopping in advance.

Your husband, if he is to be a suitable helper, should know how to operate the appliances such as the washing machine, dishwasher, and oven. He should know how to cook or prepare the meals that you have planned. And he should have attended some of the baby-care courses you attended during your pregnancy.

He should be reading this book, as well as other books on infant care and development.

Some husbands are great household managers, and some aren't. Marie found her husband was really great. "He stayed home for a week to help me and completely took over everything, so all I had to do was rest and take care of the baby and feel loved."

Elizabeth's husband turned out to make more problems than he solved. "He really tried," she said, "in fact made gourmet dinners every night. But all I wanted was toast and coffee and to be left alone."

Talk it over between yourselves.

Baby-sitters and how to choose them.

Most of the baby-sitting chores for a new baby are simple: be there when it is asleep, change diapers, feed it a bottle, burp it, and know a few tricks for when it wakes up crying. But you never know when there is going to be an emergency —a fire, an accident, an older child hurting himself—these are the times that make it important for you to choose a sitter carefully. These possible emergencies make it vital to find a sitter—at whatever age—who is coolheaded and intelligent and who has common sense.

If you are going out only when the baby and other children are asleep, then any normally responsible person is satisfactory as a sitter, whether teen-ager or adult. However, if the person will be feeding, bathing, or doing other tasks, it is best to have someone who has experience at dealing with new babies—either a mature woman who has had children of her own, or teen-agers who have had babies in their own families to care for, or someone who has taken courses in baby-sitting from the YWCA, Red Cross, or similar organization.

To find a sitter, check with friends, neighbors, and relatives. Call a baby-sitting service. Call a local college or nursing school where lists of prospects are often available.

You may also wish to try a limited responsibility sitter—someone whom you would not necessarily trust to take complete charge, but who can help with some things. A subteenager, for example, could stay with the napping baby while you run a few errands or go for a walk, or could come in to play with your older toddlers for an hour a day to give you a break.

When choosing the sitter, be sure to ask for and check references. If you have older children, be sure to introduce them to the sitter so that you can see how they get along. Agree upon the fee that you will be paying.

What the sitter expects.

The sitter should have reasonable advance notice as to when you will be needing her. You should always tell her in advance if she will be needed to stay late. You are expected to escort her home if she is young.

Try to arrive home by the time you have designated, and if you are going to be late, be courteous enough to call and say that you will be delayed.

The sitter does not expect to do household chores, although she should expect to clean up after herself. Be sure to tell her if she can fix herself coffee, a soft drink, or other snack.

Baby-sitting checklist.

The first time a person sits for you, walk her through the house, pointing out the children's rooms, where the diapers and other supplies are, what food should be prepared. You should have the baby's bottles prepared ahead of time so that the sitter only has to remove them from the refrigerator.

Each time you go out, give the sitter specific written instructions with time schedules for when you want things done. Always give her the name and telephone number of where you can be reached. Also leave the name and telephone number of the baby's doctor.

Make it clear what your rules are on food, the phone, and whether she is allowed visitors.

If you are going to have sitters frequently, it is a good idea to make several copies of all these things in writing, also including location of fuse boxes, fire extinguishers, first aid kit, and telephone numbers of relatives. It can save a great deal of time to hand copies of the instructions to your sitter as you leave, and also ensures that you will not forget to tell her anything essential.

Will the child's personality be affected by extensive day care away from the working mother?

Research on young infants indicates that personality and mental development at six months of age are independent of whether babies are cared for by their own mothers full time, or by a combination of the mother and part-time caretakers while the mother works outside the home.

Dr. Leon J. Yarrow and associates at the National Institute of Child Health and Human Development designed a method of assessing factors that affect personality development in babies.

On all of the eleven measures of stimulation that were examined, mothers scored higher than substitutes. Mothers were more likely to play and to express positive feelings toward the infants, to place toys within the baby's reach, to provide a wide selection of playthings, and to interact with the baby in a variety of ways.

However, infants cared for by mothers did not differ at six months of age in mental and personality developments from babies with part-time substitute mothers.

The importance of the father, at least to sons, emerged when Dr. Yarrow and associates applied the method to another study. Female infants, five to six months old, were not measurably affected by a lack of father interaction. In male infants, however, important measures of mental, social, and motivational development were related to how much interaction they had with their fathers. Male babies with more interaction were, at six months of age, more alert, responsive, and interested in their environment.

Dr. Yarrow speculates that the father may function to

complement stimulation by the mother and to introduce novelty into the infant's daily routine. Why only male infants seemed affected by the absence of the father is puzzling.

Although the study did not precisely explain the nature of the father's effect, it did indicate that the mother is not the sole major influence on the young infant.

Day-care centers.

There are many day-care centers in many parts of the country. A day-care center is a place where a busy or working mother can bring her infant and leave the infant for the day. The infant will be cared for by the day-care center. This is very similar to leaving the baby at the baby-sitter's house, except that in day-care centers many mothers leave many babies.

You can find out about these centers by checking the phone book yellow pages or by speaking to other mothers with young children.

The day-care center will welcome your inspection and visit; many are licensed and inspected by state governments.

The mutually beneficial trade.

Later on you may be able to work out something with someone who can baby-sit for you while you do something for them in exchange. One of our neighbors, for example, leaves her three-month-old baby once a week with an elderly but capable neighbor who enjoys the company. And in return, she does the woman's grocery shopping for her.

The baby-sitting co-op.

The co-op system has been going on for years now, just as effectively as ever. A number of mothers—usually about twenty or thirty—get together and exchange baby-sitting services. There are no fees. When someone sits for you, you pay back by sitting for someone else in the club. A list is made up of names, addresses, and telephone numbers. Each month there is a different secretary. Members call in their needs for sitting, the secretary calls members until she finds someone to take the job. And she keeps track of the number of hours owed, always calling first the women who owe the most hours so they can work them off. Daytime sitting is usually done in the sitter's house; nighttime sitting in the child's home.

You can ask around your neighborhood to see if there are such co-ops that you might join, or you might try to start one of your own. Even half a dozen people to exchange hours can make it worthwhile.

9

Physical Changes and Common Problems After Delivery— and What to Do About Them

What has happened to your body during pregnancy and delivery is fairly complex, but once you understand what has happened, you need not be mystified by it, and you will be better equipped to understand what is happening as you return to your nonpregnant state.

When you are pregnant, your estrogen and progesterone levels are high, your uterus reaches to just under your ribs, your abdomen is distended, the abdominal skin is stretched forward, and numerous internal accommodations of tissues and organs and hormones have taken place.

And in ten minutes in the delivery room the uterus empties, the hormone factory called the placenta is expelled, the abdomen and uterus contract, and a rapid succession of changes begins.

An ongoing process of changes occurs as your body begins a return to the normal, nonpregnant state. Some are visible, as are the changes in the uterus or abdomen. Some are internal and invisible, as are the changes in your hormones, your circulatory system, your muscles, and your feelings.

The physiology of becoming nonpregnant is just as complex as the physiology of becoming pregnant. And it is important for you to understand the details of this time so that you can take an active role in helping yourself to stay healthy and to ensure your health in the future.

Getting back to normal.

During pregnancy the mother's body took nine months to undergo all its changes in preparation for delivery. The return of the mother to normal occurs much more rapidly, with the greatest changes occurring during the first six weeks after delivery. This six-week period is called the *puerperium.*

Involution is the term for the changes that occur in the various organs and in the body returning to the normal, nonpregnant state. Most of the changes in involution are complete by the second or third month after delivery.

Involution actually begins as soon as the baby and placenta are delivered. Changes immediately start occurring in the uterus and abdominal wall. And soon changes also begin to take place in the skin, in the body fluid distribution, and in other parts of the body.

Simultaneously, as this involution is taking place, the breasts are undergoing changes in the opposite direction. They expand and develop in function and will not involute until nursing is either rejected by the mother or, many months later, is completed.

The uterus.

Prior to the onset of your labor you could have felt your uterus at about three finger breadths below your ribs. If you reach your hand down to feel your uterus just as soon as you are taken out of the stirrups after the delivery of the baby and the placenta, you will be able to feel the uterus as a hard lump half way between your navel and your pubic bone. Usually it will stay that way for about two days. By the third day after birth the uterus will begin to descend into the cavity of the pelvis. By the fourth or fifth day, just before going home, you will barely be able to feel the uterus one finger breadth above your pubic bone. After you're home a week you might not be able to feel it at all.

The way the uterus quickly decreases in size is astounding. At the time of delivery it weighs two pounds, one week later is down to one pound, and the week after that it weighs only three quarters of a pound. The uterus barely weighs two ounces by the time you have your postpartum checkup. That is a weight loss of about two pounds that you can really count on, whether you diet or not.

The mechanism of involution of the uterus is fairly complex. It consists of two systems. One is a system by which muscle cells actually diminish tremendously in size. Protein within the muscular cells is removed and metabolized by the body and excreted in the urine. The other mechanism is that the muscular cells of the uterus contract greatly. It is these contractions that you feel as afterpains. They are more intense during the first few days after the birth of the baby, and then they gradually diminish. But you can feel afterpains or contractions for as long as four to five weeks after the baby was born. Aspirin is sufficient to take away the pain of these afterbirth contractions. The pain is frequently intensified during nursing because the baby's sucking causes the release of a hormone called oxytocin from the pituitary gland in the mother's brain. Oxytocin is the milk-let-down hormone; it also acts as a powerful muscular stimulant to the uterus, increasing the contractile forces of involution.

Weight loss after delivery.

The average woman will lose about twelve pounds in the delivery room. The baby weighs about seven pounds, the placenta weighs about one and a half pounds, and the amniotic fluid weighs about one and a half pounds. Other fluids and some blood loss account for two pounds.

In the next week she loses about three pounds more from excretion of surplus water that was in the tissues. And two pounds is lost as the uterus reduces from two pounds to a few ounces.

Weight loss after that will be more gradual and will depend on your diet and how much you exercise.

Knowing your anatomy.

Before we talk further about the changes after delivery and advice to help you get back in shape, let's review normal female anatomy and physiology.

It is astounding how very little of their anatomy is known to most women. It will help you to take better care of your body if you know what it is really about.

The first thing to do to become acquainted with your own anatomy is to sit on the bed or on the floor, spread your legs wide, and using a hand mirror, examine yourself. Compare what you see with the diagrams following.

The hairy mound which you see as the lowest part of your abdomen is called the mons pubis. If you press against this you will feel your pubic bone running across the lower part of your abdomen.

Now follow the parts covered with pubic hair running from your mons pubis along the inner aspects of your thighs. These are the labia majora or major lips, which guard the vagina. If you spread these lips apart, you see that just within the labia majora are the labia minora, the inner lips. The labia minora meet just under your pubic bone at the clitoris, the sensitive sexual organ.

Below the clitoris is the urethral opening through which you urinate, and just below that is the vaginal opening. At the bottom of the vaginal opening you may see some remain-

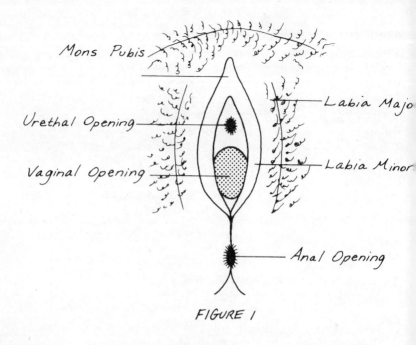

Mons Pubis

Urethal Opening

Vaginal Opening

Labia Majora

Labia Minora

Anal Opening

FIGURE 1

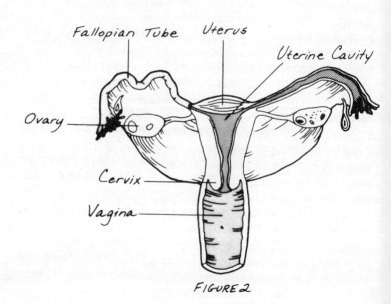

Fallopian Tube

Uterus

Uterine Cavity

Ovary

Cervix

Vagina

FIGURE 2

ing stitches that have not as yet dissolved. That is where the episiotomy was cut.

And continuing backwards, or posteriorly, is the anal opening. If you have any hemorrhoids left after delivery, they will look like red swellings protruding here.

The internal female organs are fascinating also. If you look at figure two you can see the location of the uterus and the ovaries, the internal female reproductive organs. The uterus joins the top of the vagina, which was the birth canal during your delivery.

If you lie flat on your back you can reach your hand down to feel the pubic bone. Just above the pubic bone you can feel the protuberance of your uterus until a week or ten days after delivery. After that, the uterus disappears behind the pubic bone as it shrinks down by involuting.

The abdomen after delivery.

If you stand sideways in front of a full-length mirror the day after you deliver, you might be rather disappointed. Your tummy will look as if you are still five months pregnant, and in some people it will look like they are seven or eight months pregnant. There is a brown line extending from your navel to your pubic bone called the "linea negra." And in most people there will also be some increased pigmentation of the skin below and around the navel. It looks like you haven't bathed in a while.

Will exercises help my abdominal bulge?

Not at this time, because the abdominal wall has to involute in the natural fashion before you can increase its tone by exercise. This means that you have to be patient and wait for the stretched muscle fibers of the anterior abdominal wall to reduce their size and to shrink down. Then exercises definitely help. By the time you go home, a sidelong glance in the mirror will show just that you look about four months pregnant. It may take one or two more weeks before you begin to look not pregnant at all!

Your waist size will continue to go down also, but usually it will be one inch larger after having delivered a baby than it was before you were pregnant, even after involution of the abdominal wall and your exercises have been completed. However, you don't add an inch with every baby, but merely lose that inch once.

At four weeks postpartum, the musculature has shortened as much as it will shorten naturally. At this point exercises will be very beneficial in tightening and firming.

Will the skin discoloration go away?

The brown line that you have after birth will gradually fade away until it's finally gone a few months after the baby is born. Similarly, the increased brown pigmentation and freckling of the lower abdominal wall will also gradually fade and disappear within three months.

The stretch marks that occur in some people and that might be brownish or reddish are called striae. These striae will gradually lose their color and will shrink, but usually they will continue to remain forever as small scars that occurred from the stretching of the connective tissue of the abdominal wall skin. But there is a trick to getting rid of striae, which may not make them disappear completely, but which will make them almost invisible. The trick is to get two really deep suntans in one year—a good excuse to take a vacation in the Caribbean. The sun and the ultraviolet rays cause these scars to shrink down a great deal so that the striae may actually become mere hairline marks, almost invisible.

Other skin changes from pregnancy.

Changes in your hormones can affect your skin in strange ways. For instance, you may develop pigments during pregnancy with dark patches on the face (called the "mask of pregnancy"). The increase in pigment also increases the darkness of already dark areas in the genital area, around the nipples, at the navel, and in a straight line down the middle of the abdomen. If you have any recent scars, they may darken also. Most of this coloring returns to normal within a few weeks after delivery. If the patches on your face remain prominent, your doctor can give you a lotion to lessen them.

In many women the palms of the hands get very red. This too will pass.

Another strange skin happening is small, pinhead-size bumps, called skin tags. They usually show up on the breasts, the neck, or under the arms. Usually they do not disappear after delivery, but get bigger with each pregnancy. They really don't bother anything, but your doctor can remove them after pregnancy, if you want him to.

About two out of three women also get "spiders," little elevated skin markings with branches going out like legs. They are overgrown ends of tiny arteries and are bright red. They usually disappear within two months after delivery. Any that persist can be destroyed with a very fine electric needle.

Hairiness on unusual sites may also occur from hormone changes. The new hairs usually shed within three months postpartum. If they persist after that, they may be removed by electrolysis.

What about hair loss?

Most women go through a period of hair loss from the scalp about four to six months after the baby is born. It is frequently frightening; often large clumps of hair come out in the comb or brush.

This hair loss is normal and only lasts for a short time. It is due to the fact that hair that grew during pregnancy has a shorter life expectancy than your usual hair.

If the hair loss lasts for more than one month, you should consult a dermatologist who will examine you to be sure that you don't have a scalp illness.

Vaginal and perineal care at home.

You can ease healing and help yourself feel better by standing in a warm shower and letting warm water run over your backside and bathe the stitch area. This stimulates blood flow and will help healing. In addition, after you return home, you can take baths in very shallow water. These are called sitz baths. The water is kept no deeper than *two or three inches* so that it will not enter the uppermost part of the vagina where it might enter the uterus and cause infection.

Stitches in your perineum heal quickly, and usually healing is completed by the fifth day. This means that you will probably be without stitch pain by the fifth day, but it doesn't mean that you should test the stitches. The tissues won't achieve strength sufficient for intercourse until about four weeks after delivery.

Other ways to soothe soreness of the perineum are by applying anesthetic lotions or sprays, using a heat lamp, and taking aspirin or other pain-killers.

Hemorrhoids.

Because of the pushing that you do to help the delivery of the baby, and with the great pressures that the baby's head and body exert as they pass through the birth canal, hemorrhoids frequently pop out during the time of delivery. Hemorrhoids are actually dilated blood vessels that enlarge to bulbous swellings around the anus. They sometimes hurt more than stitches. There is no specific treatment. You might try an anesthetic ointment to take away the acute pain or you might try standing in a warm shower, because the heat will help the dilated blood vessels. Wiping with witch hazel will also help ease the pain. But time usually helps hemorrhoids more than anything, and they are usually gone ten days after the birth of the baby.

It is very important to keep your bowel movement fairly soft, as a constipated stool will rub against the hemorrhoids and irritate them further. Drinking three quarts of water daily is the best way to keep from being constipated.

Vaginal discharge.

The vaginal discharge after delivery, called lochia, has a bright red color for the first three or four days, then becomes pale pink. Lochia is not menstruation, but it is somewhat like a very heavy period for the first day or two after delivery, then gradually subsides. You should wear sanitary pads, not tampons.

There is no way of predicting when your lochia will end

and you can't even judge it from day to day. It characteristically gets less and less and usually by the time you are going home from the hospital two or three sanitary pads a day are sufficient.

Sometimes it will stop totally for a day or two and then resume almost like a fresh period. Usually lochia subsides within four or five weeks after the baby is born, but sometimes it can continue lightly for about six to eight weeks.

If the lochia stops about a week or two after you have delivered and then suddenly seems to increase and gush again, it usually is a tip that you are working too hard, that your uterus has relaxed, and that the involution has regressed, allowing some of the blood vessels that were closed to open up again. This should be a sign to take more rest and to reevaluate some of your activities.

Later discharge.

Even when you are not pregnant, the vagina has a sticky mucus present, but usually the amount is small. During pregnancy and after your postpartum bleeding stops, you will still often notice a white, sticky discharge. It merely means that the vaginal passage is still heavily lubricated.

If you suddenly have more discharge than usual, if it becomes yellow or green or frothy, or if you have itching of the genital area, tell your doctor. It may be an infection and need treatment.

Don't use douches unless your doctor orders them.

When does true menstruation begin?

The time varies tremendously. If the woman does not breast-feed, the menstrual period usually reappears within six to eight weeks after delivery. In the woman who nurses, there is even more irregularity, and the menses may return any time from the second to the eighteenth month, with the average at about five months.

If you are nursing, you usually won't menstruate during the time you are nursing, although some people defy the average and begin to menstruate about two months after the birth, even though still nursing. The variabilities are enormous, with most people not menstruating while they are nursing, and some not beginning to menstruate until six to eight months after they have completed nursing. This doesn't mean that the menstrual flow is building up inside of you at all. What it means is that it is taking you that much longer to produce the necessary hormones to build up the lining of the uterus to a point where it will be ready to slough off and come out as menstrual flow.

That first period after childbirth will be quite variable. In some people there will be rapid production of hormones, causing a rapid growth of the lining of the uterus, then ovulation, followed by a sloughing of that lining. Others will have a very slow output of hormone, causing excessive thickening of the uterus lining. By the time ovulation finally occurs, the sloughing off of this very thick lining can cause a very heavy and scary menstrual period.

If your first period seems particularly heavy, go to bed and count the number of pads you are using. You can safely use a pad per hour for six or seven hours without running into danger, but if the heavy flow of a pad an hour continues longer than six or seven hours, or if you start to have to change a pad every half an hour, you should call your doctor right away.

With future menstrual periods, the amount of bleeding may be more or less than you had before you were pregnant, and the periods may still be irregular, as though your hormone cycles haven't quite zeroed in on their adjustment yet.

Passing clots of blood.

Rosemary T. had been home about a week from the hospital when one morning on getting up and going to the bathroom she felt a huge clot of blood pass from her vagina. It was as large as a bowel movement. She was frantic, afraid something terrible had happened.

Actually this is more common than generally believed. If there is some bleeding and heavy discharge while you are sleeping on your back, the blood accumulates in a pocket in the vagina, forms a loose, large clot, and then comes out when you awake and stand up.

This occurrence is not dangerous, but it does require your attention and evaluation. In order to tell the difference between a clot due to accumulated blood and a clot due to rapid excessive bleeding, keep a pad count while you are up with moderate activity. Follow the guideline that if it seems as much as a normal period you can stay with normal activities. And if it is more, you should get in bed and periodically change your pad to check on the blood loss.

Remember, you can safely use a pad per hour for about six hours. Call your doctor if you are using more than that.

Sweating and hot flashes.

Quite a bit of hormone function is related to the placenta, so that when the placenta, or afterbirth, is delivered, there is a diminished production of hormones in the body. Because of this, hot flashes can occur just like those that occur in the menopause. These are characterized by attacks of profuse sweating which can cause you to soak through your bed clothing. Actually, sweating is quite helpful because it helps to mobilize some of the edema fluid and get it out of your system. In addition, during the first day or two in bed, the urine volume is increased as edema fluid is mobilized and leaves the body. If you are sweating a great deal, be sure to measure your temperature so that you know it is not infection and fever causing the sweating.

To feel fresh after sweating so much, simply wash more and shower frequently.

Itching.

About one out of five women feels an intense itching of the abdomen during or after pregnancy, apparently due to stretching of the abdominal wall. Putting a lotion of phenol and camphor in olive oil and lime water on the skin will help. Sometimes stronger lotions with corticosteroids are needed.

If you have itching all over your body, you should tell your doctor about it right away. It could be an allergic reaction or an upset in liver function that will mean a change in diet is necessary.

What can I do for heartburn?

If you avoid greasy or fried foods, you can generally prevent heartburn, which, by the way, has nothing to do with your heart, but is caused by excess acid in your stomach. Antacids, either liquid or tablets, will help, but be sure they are the kind that do not contain sodium. Do not use sodium bicarbonate (baking soda).

Can I do anything for constipation?

People who have never been bothered in their entire lives with constipation often are troubled with it during pregnancy and the postpartum period. You can take milk of magnesia two or three times a week and usually solve the problem.

Or help avoid constipation by adding more bulky food to your diet. Also eat plenty of fruits and vegetables and drink plenty of water. If necessary, eat a few raisins or prunes or drink prune juice. If you still have trouble, check with your doctor about taking other laxatives. Two or three bowel movements per week are sufficient. There is no need to have a bowel movement every day—however your body works best is fine.

What if I get dizzy and feel faint?

If you stand in one place for a long time, your blood tends to pool in your legs and pelvis. This reduces blood available for your heart to pump to the brain. The next thing you know, especially if the room is hot, you've swooned gently to the floor. If you feel dizziness coming on, sit or lie down. Sometimes walking or contracting your leg muscles will help, but it's better to sit down.

What can I do about always feeling tired?

Remember how absolutely exhausted you were during the first three months of pregnancy? Your head would start to nod in the middle of the afternoon, or you'd fall asleep on the couch after dinner. It's the same way for many weeks after you come home from the hospital.

So put your feet up and relax several times a day. Even if it's only for ten or fifteen minutes. Take a nap every afternoon. Quit working *before* you get tired. So the beds don't get made. You need the rest now so that months later you'll have more energy.

Should I take iron pills?

Anemia can cause excessive fatigue. When you go to your doctor for regular checkups during pregnancy, he may do a blood count to see if you are anemic or not. There are many causes for anemia, but most of the time it is due to an iron deficiency, and your doctor will have you take some iron pills. A glass of orange juice every day will also help to increase iron absorption and to stimulate production of red blood cells.

There is some degree of iron deficiency in 70 to 80 percent of all women, whether pregnant or not. And even if not anemic before pregnancy, most women develop some degree of anemia sometime during the course of their pregnancy.

If a routine hemoglobin test shows your hemoglobin levels are low, you should take ferrous iron in the simplest and least expensive form available. The usual prescription is a total of one hundred milligrams of iron per day in divided doses two to three times per day. There is no point in increasing the dosage, because it cannot be absorbed any faster.

Iron levels usually fall until the eighth month of pregnancy, then rise, then drop again in the postpartum period.

If anemia is severe or there is no response to iron, there may be other causes. Your doctor will want to check for sickle cell, megaloblastic, or other anemia.

How much rest do I need?

Obtaining enough regular rest is the most important single thing you can do to put yourself back onto the road to healthy physical shape.

Bustling around with too much work and not enough sleep can cause menstrual troubles later. And in the immediate postpartum period—the first few weeks—it can interfere with involution with resultant delayed hemorrhage or infection. Insufficient rest can cause delay of healing and recovery to health, and because of the constant fatigue you feel, it can cause you to be irritable and tense, and can diminish your milk supply.

So the number one rule for taking care of yourself and getting back better than ever is to get enough rest. Definite periods of rest. Not whenever you can after the housework is done, but definite, regularly scheduled periods of rest, twice every day, no matter whether the housework is done or not. One nap in the morning and one in the afternoon.

After one month you can drop down to one nap a day if you no longer feel tired in late morning. But keep that afternoon nap for at least another month. And that means actually sleeping, not just with your feet up or reading.

Increased urination.

Increased frequency and urgency often occur during the postpartum period, especially in the first week. This is because so much fluid has been retained during pregnancy. Now your body is getting rid of it. There is nothing you can do about it except to remember to go to the bathroom before you leave the house and develop a sense of humor. It is normal and will go away. If you have sudden frequency of urination after you come home, or have a burning sensation during urination, call your doctor.

What about burning during urination?

Burning during urination is a frequent complaint in the postpartum period and it is usually not due to infection. During the birth process the baby's head presses very strongly against the lower bladder and the urethra. As a result, the bladder walls and urethra are swollen, inflamed, and sensitive. The inflamed linings are particularly sensitive to concentrated urine, which causes burning with urination.

The burning feeling is a signal that you should increase your fluid intake and be sure that you are drinking at least three quarts of liquid per day. And at least two of those three quarts should be water. Your urine should be so dilute that it is almost clear in color.

Usually, within twenty-four hours of starting your increased fluid intake schedule, your burning should pass. If it persists longer than that or if you have a temperature above 100 degrees Fahrenheit, you should call the doctor.

What can I do for low back pain?

During pregnancy, the center of gravity of the body shifts forward, causing most women to stand in a sway back position, which puts stress and strain on the back and legs. Often low back pain persists after delivery.

Try to stand with your seat tucked under. Pelvis tilt exercises will help (see Chapter 11.)

Also, it sometimes helps to straighten your back out, standing firmly against a wall or door, or lying flat on the floor, pushing your back down to touch the floor.

You may want to use a maternity girdle to help ease the strain on back muscles. And use low-heeled, well-made shoes for a while longer to give you better balance.

Should I wear a girdle?

While we can give you many reasons to wear a brassiere, the decision whether or not to wear a girdle is really a matter of personal preference. Some women feel more comfortable wearing a girdle. It neither helps nor hinders the process of involution.

But girdles do help the back pain of pregnancy and the persistence of this pain after pregnancy. You can understand this if you consider the two reasons for back pain in pregnancy.

One cause is the mechanical effect of the increasing weight of the pregnant uterus causing a forward force for which a postural compensation is made, thus straining the sacroiliac and lower vertebral joints. This is corrected by delivering the baby and returning the forces on the joints to normal.

The second cause of back pain is the result of the relaxation of the ligaments and capsules of the joints due to the effects of the hormones of pregnancy. The increased elasticity around the joints allows excessive movements, which cause stresses and pain. While the hormone levels drop rapidly once the placenta is out of your body, the affected ligaments may take a few weeks' time to return to a less elastic state.

A girdle helps pain due to this cause because it acts like an external limiting ligament, preventing excessive flexions and movements of the back joints.

If you get cramps in your legs.

Leg cramps usually represent a calcium deficiency. The cramps are due to the fact that the calcium of your muscles is being depleted. This does not mean that you need more milk. It is a fallacy that milk is necessary for calcium needs in pregnancy. Calcium in milk is present as calcium phosphate and will be excreted by your kidneys.

If you have leg cramps, increase your calcium intake by taking calcium lactate tablets, or by eating more meat or cheese. And for the acute cramps, leg massage and a heating pad will help.

What can I do for varicose veins?

The bulging out of veins during pregnancy occurs because of the increased blood volume of pregnancy and the resultant increase in pressure of the blood in the veins. The mechanical contribution of the growing uterus also increases the pressure in the veins, particularly below the waist. There is a hereditary factor also, with some women being more likely to develop varicose veins than others.

Varicose veins may occur in the legs or near the opening to the vagina. Wear elastic support stockings for the first, a sanitary pad for the second. Don't ever wear elastic garters or roll your stockings at the top. This acts as a tourniquet and reduces returning circulation in the legs. Wear a maternity girdle or maternity garter belt, or nothing. Put supporting stockings on in the morning before you leave your bed and before the veins have a chance to fill. Elevate your feet several times a day to help drain the blood. Do the leg and foot exercises described in Chapter 11.

Usually varicose veins disappear, or at least improve greatly, after delivery. If they are still a problem, they can be treated surgically or by injection.

Sometimes groups of veins will also enlarge and swell in the lower end of the rectum. They are called hemorrhoids or piles. Your doctor can give you compresses for these. Suppositories containing a local anesthetic will ease any pain. Particularly avoid constipation if you have hemorrhoids, since straining makes them worse.

Mouth problems.

Some women have swelling of the gums during pregnancy, and sometimes the gums become discolored and bleed easily. The condition may persist after delivery. Be especially careful to follow good oral hygiene, and most of the problem will disappear in a few weeks. Mild astringents and mouthwashes help. If you get sores or the swelling interferes with chewing, consult your doctor or dentist.

Women have said for a long time that they get more cavities when they are pregnant, but there has never been any scientific evidence to show this. However, it is a good idea to see a dentist during the postpartum period.

What can I do for painful breast engorgement?

Whether you have nursed or not, breast engorgement can be very painful with the swelling and inflammation that occurs in the breasts when they are filling with milk.

Wear a firm bra day and night to limit the swelling. Take aspirin for the inflammation, which you will notice as warmth and tenderness; the breasts might even turn reddish or become flushed. To further reduce inflammation, make two ice caps by putting ice cubes in a towel and applying the towels with ice to your breasts. Leave your bra on for its mechanical effect in containing the swelling.

Painful engorgement rarely lasts for over twenty-four hours. It can also be relieved by nursing.

Should I wear any special bra?

During the postpartum period, whether you are nursing or not, you should wear a bra day and night. The bra serves to support the breasts, which are heavier than usual at this time and tend to pull excessively at their supporting ligaments, which come from the clavicles. In addition, the bra serves as a constraint to limit sudden and excessive volume increases in the breasts due to water retention associated with the rapid hormone changes of this period.

If you are nursing, there are nursing bras that have drop fronts to enable you to feed the baby without having to remove your bra.

Is there any permanent change in the breast from pregnancy?

There is great individual variation in how breasts change due to pregnancy. In some women there are no changes whatsoever; others become totally different, sometimes better, and sometimes not.

For the most part, the breasts of women who breast-feed their babies become firmer than before, particularly if they take care to wear a bra day and night while pregnant and during the nursing period.

When should I call my doctor?

You should feel free to call your doctor whenever the thought occurs to you that you should speak to him. Sometimes it is more important to call him with a worry or fear that is troubling you than with an illness. This is a time when you will have periods of heightened sensitivity. Rather than stewing over a fear or an apprehension, call his office.

You will of course be seeing your doctor for your four- or six-week checkup, and you will certainly save some questions until then.

The following are situations in which you should call your doctor:

1. Pain and redness in the breast, accompanied by fever.

2. Any unusual persistent pain. (However, a sharp pain can occur momentarily during your activities, and you lose nothing by lying down for a few moments to see if the pain leaves.)

3. Fever or chills with temperature over 100 degrees Fahrenheit. Incidentally, oral temperatures are always sufficient at home, you need not take your rectal temperature. Wait at least five minutes after you have eaten or had any liquids before you take your temperature.

4. Numbness or blurring of vision that lasts for more than half an hour.

5. Severe headache that persists after taking two aspirin tablets and lying down to nap.

6. Excessive vaginal bleeding. Apply the criteria we discussed previously about measuring pads per hour, but don't wait at all if it is gushing.

7. If something is worrying you or if you feel depressed.

10

How to Succeed
at Breast-Feeding

In Evanston, Illinois, every day a two-woman team of volunteers jumps into a station wagon and makes the rounds of several houses, collecting breast milk from donors who have pumped their milk into collection jars. This milk is then distributed to premature babies or other infants who very much need breast milk but whose mothers for one reason or another are not able to supply it.

There are nearly one hundred breast milk banks in the United States, and even more in Europe. They are an ongoing testimonial to how important doctors think breast milk is to newborn infants.

We hope that you will breast-feed your baby. It is the best thing for him and the best thing for you.

If you decide that you will do so, this chapter will tell you how to succeed easily without fussing and fuming. It's better if you do breast-feed, but you can also raise your baby successfully with formula feedings.

Why is it better for the baby to breast-feed?

Many studies of infant development have shown that babies who have been breast-fed get sick less often and less seriously than babies who were not breast-fed.

One study, for example, showed that infants who had not been breast-fed had four times more respiratory infections in later years. And the non-breast-fed babies had twenty times more diarrhea, twenty-two times more miscellaneous infections, eight times more eczema, twenty-one times more asthma, twenty-seven times more hayfever, eleven times more surgery for tonsils and adenoids, four times more ear problems, eleven times more hospital admissions, and eight times more physician house calls.

It's obviously well worth the effort to breast-feed.

Why is mother's milk better than formula?

Human milk is composed of substances that are not foreign to the baby and so do not cause allergies. Mother's milk also contains antibodies against infections; these are believed to be carried to the baby and so protect the baby more fully against germs.

Human milk, in contrast to other formulas, is germ-free with no need for sterilization. It is easier to digest, it causes fewer intestinal upsets, and it contains more iron and vitamins.

A breast-fed baby has less difficulty getting up bubbles, since he usually swallows less air because the delivery system is so specialized.

Cow's milk does not have the proper acidity for the baby's stomach and intestines, and the minerals of cow's milk are far too concentrated for the baby. The baby's tiny kidneys cannot handle large amounts of minerals during the first few months of life. Cow's milk is subjected to many modifications in the production of bottled formula, and then it is but an approximation of the baby's needs.

What are the emotional advantages to the baby?

There is experimental evidence that the newborn baby's security is closely related to skin-to-skin contact with the mother. Cuddling the baby against a clothed arm and body of the mother during feedings is not enough.

The temporal lobe of the newborn's brain is relatively well developed at birth and is associated with smell differentiation. There is evidence that the baby can differentiate the mother by the smell of her skin.

In addition, most psychologists believe that until three or four months of age the baby considers the mother's breasts as an extension of itself. This feeling of expansiveness of self is tied to developing feelings of security.

Does breast-feeding have any advantages for the mother?

Definitely. Mothers who breast-feed have less bleeding after delivery, get back in shape sooner, and feel fit faster. Their breasts become firmer.

Statistics of breast-feeding suggest that mothers who breast-feed are less likely to develop breast cancer in future years. (One study puts the chances at one in twenty-five for women who have not breast-fed and one in one hundred twenty-five for those who have nursed a baby for six months.)

Breast-feeding does great things for getting your reproductive system back in order too. For example, during the first few weeks of nursing you will be aware of contractions of your uterus as your baby nurses. This is one specific sign of how nursing makes your uterus contract down to its usual size quickly. In addition, the vaginal discharge slows down faster in the nursing mother.

And of course breast-feeding, as you cuddle your new baby to you and feel its warmth and are able to nourish it from your own body, gives you a marvelous feeling of love and closeness to your new child. It probably does more to make you feel instantly motherly than any other single thing you can do.

On the practical side, it is tremendously convenient. When you are stuck in traffic on a freeway for three hours with a crying, hungry baby, you'll be thankful you can open your shirt and make the baby happy.

Even the shyest mother learns that she can nurse without exposing herself. It is so easy to drape a towel over a nursing baby and to feel totally secluded at that very private time in your lives together.

It is easier to do this on a plane than to wait for a stewardess to stop mixing martinis to warm the bottle. In fact one mother reports of a long, cross-country air trip in which the stewardess even refused to put a baby's bottle on ice to keep cool because it would use up ice needed for drinks!

How will nursing affect my dieting after I have the baby?

Breast-feeding provides an excellent shortcut to weight loss. The breast-fed baby takes about six hundred to seven hundred calories a day from his mother by about the fourth week of life. This means that if you follow a sixteen hundred calories a day diet (certainly a generous diet by any standards) you will have a net caloric intake for yourself of only a thousand calories.

As long as your water intake is at least three quarts a day and you are in good protein balance and take your vitamins, the milk quality will be fine. And the best news: you will lose at least two pounds per week this way.

What to do during pregnancy to get ready for breast-feeding.

Some people recommend various nipple exercises to prepare for breast-feeding, but these are actually unnecessary. Breast-feeding is a natural phenomenon and the breasts are ready at the time of birth, even if the child is born early.

Are there some women who cannot breast-feed their babies?

Almost every woman is physically equipped to do it. No matter how flat chested you are, no matter how small your nipples, no matter how unmotherly you look or feel, your equipment is perfectly satisfactory for nursing a baby. The woman who does not have sufficient breast tissue to nurse adequately is very rare.

*I want to nurse my baby, but I'm a little nervous about it
—what can I do?*

First, talk to your doctor about it. He can give you a great
deal of encouragement. Remember it is the most natural
thing in the world, and even if you have never held a baby
in your arms in your whole life, you can still do it. Think of
all the benefits it will bring to your baby, and you. Talk to
a mother who has breast-fed her babies, or even better, talk
to a mother who is nursing her baby now. Get her to demon-
strate the procedure to you. She will surely tell you about
how easy it is and how pleased she is with doing it.

You may also want to join or visit the local chapter of the
La Leche League, an organization formed to encourage
breast-feeding. The league helps women who want to do it
but aren't sure of themselves. Their national address is La
Leche League International, 9606 Franklin Avenue, Franklin Park, Illinois 60131, but the chances are that one of their
chapters is listed right in your local telephone book.

And you know you don't really have to make the decision
ahead of time. Once your baby is in your arms, needing love,
food, and care, you may instantly feel, "Of course I'm going
to nurse him!"

If you run into opposition.

As satisfying as breast-feeding can be for both mother and
baby, only about one out of four mothers in the United States
breast-feeds her baby. The percentage is closer to four of five
mothers who are college graduates, and the percentage is
much much higher in Europe and other countries where it
is taken for granted that babies will be breast-fed.

Astonishingly enough, despite the known advantages for
both mother and baby, many physicians simply do not encourage their patients to breast-feed. Medical schools and
medical textbooks spend much more time talking about artificial feeding and prescribing formulas than about breast-
feeding. Some doctors don't want to spend the time to encourage mothers to breast-feed. Others consider it their job
to get a healthy baby into the world, and the mother's job to

make decisions about how she is going to feed her baby.

Nurses, too, often busy with more than they can handle in understaffed hospitals, simply don't want to put in the time and trouble to give advice to mothers nursing for the first time.

However, most modern obstetrical units in the hospitals of today have programs in the hospital to help the mother with breast-feeding before she leaves for home with her newborn.

If the doctors and nurses you come in contact with are not enthusiastic over breast-feeding, don't be discouraged. It *is* best. It is *not* difficult; in fact, it is the easiest, most natural thing in the world, and for most of man's history has been the *only* way. Go ahead and do it!

Sometimes husbands oppose breast-feeding. Your husband may worry that it will affect your shape or that it will interfere with social engagements or with his time alone with you. He may not recognize that his objections may reflect the natural jealous feelings that he must deal with.

Involve him by sharing your enthusiasm with him and by making him a part of the rational decisions that lead you to breast-feeding.

Friends and neighbors may express negative remarks also. Ignore them. Run your own life. They may just be feeling guilty because *they* didn't breast-feed when they had children.

You may also feel pushed by your children clamoring for attention and care, by housework piling up screaming to be done. Resist. No matter how much work there is, relax, get that nap every day, and spend that peaceful time nursing your baby.

Mothers-in-law and mothers too can try to discourage you, either directly or by subtle means. Very few new mothers can succeed in breast-feeding with a mother-in-law living in the home who is hostile to the concept. No mother can compete with her daughter's mothering when that daughter is nursing her new baby. If you sense hostility, discuss the issue, and help your mother-in-law or mother define her new role as a grandmother.

One woman's story.

Cynthia C. was a perfectly competent accountant, but she had no self-confidence when it came to nursing and she had the added problem of a mother who was not enthusiastic about it.

"When it came to feeding him," she told us, "I didn't even know how to start. I really didn't have confidence. I remember when he was a week old he was crying a lot after nursing, and I was nursing him every two hours, and each feeding was lasting about an hour and a half, and I was a wreck. I was tired and I was worried and I didn't think that I could nurse. I can remember talking to my mother and I would sit there with this cracked voice about to break up in hysterics and I would say, 'I don't understand it; I'm just feeding him constantly.' Maybe if she had encouraged me . . . I don't know. I hate to say this, but I really think that deep down inside maybe she resented the fact that I was nursing. My grandmother, a baby nurse, insisted that my milk wasn't rich enough. She said I should eat lots of ice cream. I was panicky. I called up the pediatrician who I had only met in the hospital and told him I was thinking of stopping. 'Evidently I don't have enough milk for him. If I change to formula, what should I do?' He told me. I really wanted him to say, 'Don't change, you can do it.'

"That's when I called you. It was like a tranquilizer. I felt like a new person. You told me, 'You can do it, I know that you can do it.' "

Sometimes just finding that one person to encourage you can make all the difference in the world.

How does the baby actually get the milk?

The baby doesn't really suck as one would from a straw. It milks the breast by a combined action of thrusting its tongue out under the nipple and drawing the nipple back into its mouth, while at the same time squeezing down with its gums on the areolar area to force the milk out. In response to this action by the baby, the muscles of the milk ducts contract and actually squirt milk into the baby's mouth.

What should the milk look like?

The first milk that comes in is actually colostrum, a yellowish fluid that is rich in protein and antibodies. But this fluid is not really a good source of nourishment. It is all the baby needs in the first day or so after delivery, however, because the baby is born with excess fluids in its body to tide it over until your milk comes in. The milk actually comes in two to three days after delivery, gradually at first, then increasing in supply as the production is stimulated by the milk being taken by the baby. This milk has a thin consistency and a bluish color much like that of skimmed milk.

When should I begin nursing?

Right away. Either on the delivery table or on the first day when the baby is brought to you. The baby won't get anything from it at first, and it really doesn't need anything then, but the stimulation of the nursing will help to start the milk flowing.

If you are at all nervous about this first encounter, try to make it take place under quiet, peaceful, and private circumstances.

The first nursing period.

You need a few minutes in preparation.

First wash your hands thoroughly with soap and water, and cleanse the breasts and nipples with water. Hop into bed, get comfortably propped up on your pillows, fold back a corner of the sheet to make a clean place for the baby, and relax.

When the nurse brings the baby to you, cuddle it in the crook of your arm and enjoy its beauty. Stick the nipple into the baby's mouth, holding your breast in such a way that you don't block the child's nose. It may voraciously lunge at the breast, or—more likely—the baby will lie there half-asleep as if it hasn't the slightest idea what to do. So that makes two of you—you're even!

Stroke its cheek and mouth—that will usually stimulate the baby to open its mouth. Move your breast around a little

—the baby will eventually get the idea.

To prevent sore or cracked nipples during the first days, limit nursing to one minute for each breast at any one time. If baby is still hungry, let him go back to each breast for extra time, up to five or ten minutes total on each breast if he wants it the first day.

Again, relax on this first encounter. It doesn't really matter whether the baby gets anything substantial on this first feeding.

Care of your breasts and nipples.

Be sure your nursing bra gives support to the breasts and is not too tight. Wear it for sleep as well as by day for maximum support. Take out any plastic or rubberized sections.

Wash your breasts during your shower using warm water and a soft, clean washcloth. Do not use soap. Washing with soap, especially to excess, removes natural oils that protect the skin from drying and cracking.

Expose your breasts to the air whenever possible. At night, for example, you might sleep with the flaps of your nursing bra down.

Apply cream or ointment to your nipples after every feeding, making sure that your nipples are dry before applying creams. Good preparations include Masse cream, A&D ointment, lanolin, cocoa butter, and Nivea cream.

While in the hospital, use the reading lamp above your bed to give your breasts a heat treatment. Focus the light above your breasts for ten to fifteen minutes, two or three times a day. You may wish to continue this at home.

Be sure baby has the whole nipple and most of the areola (brown area around the nipple) in his mouth, for proper sucking. Do not allow your baby to pull on the nipple when you take him from the breast. You must break the suction he makes with his mouth.

Do not be discouraged if your nipples become sore during your first few days of nursing. Continue to nurse, and your breasts will toughen up.

Consult your doctor if any local area of redness or tenderness occurs.

If leaking occurs, and you wish to protect clothing from milk stains, use a nursing pad (one without plastic), a gauze pad, or a clean handkerchief. Change to a clean bra daily.

If your nipples are flat or inverted, use a breast shield, which may help the baby in drawing out your nipple.

Temporary engorgement and what to do about that.

Your breasts may become engorged, full and swollen, on the third or fourth day after delivery. This is partly due to the beginning of heavy milk production and partly to swelling of breast tissue itself and increased blood flow into the breast veins. The discomfort lasts only twenty-four to forty-eight hours, until the milk begins to flow freely. A warm shower or hot towels placed over the breasts will often sooth them—and you—and help relaxation. If they become painful during this time you may also use ice packs or take an aspirin or other analgesic. If engorgement becomes really bad, your doctor can give you some oxytocin just before the baby nurses. Oxytocin is the milk-let-down hormone that is also produced naturally during breast-feeding. It also acts directly on uterine muscle to cause the contractions you may feel as cramps while nursing.

What to do before each feeding.

Wash your hands with soap and water, just as you did for the first nursing period. Have clean fingernails. Wash your breasts with warm water. Get yourself and your baby comfortable in a bed or a chair. Supporting the baby with a pillow on your lap may be helpful. Try different positions until you find the one that best suits both of you. Sometimes it is easier to nurse if you lie on your abdomen with your breasts extending downward to the baby's mouth.

Have a table nearby so that you can keep on it something to drink, tissues, or anything else you may need during the feeding.

Relax.

During feeding.

Hold the baby close to your body so its cheek touches your nipple, thus stimulating the rooting reflex. The baby may try side-to-side motions with his head; this causes the nipple to become erect and makes it easier for him to grasp it. You may cause the same effect by stimulating the nipple with your fingers.

Your baby may locate the nipple for itself and begin to suck. If not, grasp your nipple at its base and insert the entire nipple and some of the surrounding dark tissue into the baby's mouth.

Allow some breathing space for the baby, especially if your breasts are very full. Simply compress the breast slightly beneath the baby's nose. If you are lying down on your side, you can usually pull its legs close to you and angle its body enough to keep its nose free.

When taking the baby off the breast, break the suction first. Gently press the breast away from the corner of its mouth with your finger or pull its mouth down on one side or gently hold its nose shut for a few seconds.

Other tips on nursing.

This is a time to lavish attention on yourself. Try to avoid anything that will make you nervous, anxious, angry, or tired. Make sure you get enough rest. *It is absolutely essential that you get a nap every day,* preferably two. Spend most of the first three days at home in bed. Let somebody else do the housework. More than anything else, to produce lots of milk you need rest.

In the first few days, and even later, allow the baby to control the number of daily feedings, even though they come every two or three hours instead of the artificially specified four hours.

Don't worry if your baby doesn't seem to be satisfied at first. Milk always comes slowly in the beginning. Relax. The milk will increase as your baby needs more.

A glass of wine a half hour before nursing will help your milk flow freely.

To encourage production of milk, nurse at every feeding the first few days, including the night feedings.

On the day you deliver and the day after, nurse five minutes on each breast. By starting slowly, and then gradually increasing feeding time, you may prevent sore and cracked nipples.

On the second day after delivery, let the baby have five minutes on each breast, then go back for an extra turn on each if he wishes.

On the third day after delivery, your milk may begin to come in. Nurse five minutes on one side and five minutes on the other. And from now on let the baby have as much extra time on the second breast as it wants. Usually thirty minutes of nursing provides as much nourishment and oral stimulation as infants require.

Continue to alternate the breasts with which you begin feedings to provide equal stimulation. Keep tabs with a safety pin fastened to the bra of the next one to be started with. And always switch the baby to the other breast after five minutes on the first breast so that the baby gets the maximum amount of milk without getting tired and so that your breasts don't get sore.

Burp your baby before offering the second breast and after feeding is completed. The "over-the-shoulder," "sitting-on-your-lap," and "over-the-knee" methods are all effective. Remember, breast-fed babies may burp less than bottle-fed babies; some babies do not burp at all.

Avoid becoming overtired. Breast milk tends to diminish if you become overtired or upset. If possible, get some help with household chores. You absolutely must take naps. Nurse your baby when it appears to be hungry, usually anywhere from every two and a half to four hours. But don't wake the baby up to feed, and let the baby begin sleeping through the night as soon as possible.

Since some medications may appear in your breast milk, consult your doctor before taking *any* medications while breast-feeding.

Bowel movements

Breast-fed babies have frequent, loose bowel movements. Early in life, movements are dark green or black. Later they become yellow and may be quite liquid in consistency. Your baby may have as many as eight to ten bowel movements a day; quite often they occur during or after meals. On the other hand, he may have only one bowel movement every few days. In either event, don't worry about it.

Inverted nipples

If you have inversion of the nipples—that is, if they stick in instead of out—the condition will usually correct itself automatically during pregnancy. But if after delivery there is still inversion, you can make nursing easier by wearing a nursing shield. It consists of a rubber nursing nipple attached to a plastic funnel that is applied over the breast, which the infant grabs and sucks. The sucking action gradually pulls out the mother's nipple so that it protrudes properly.

The let-down reflex.

The breast tissue may be filled with milk, but the milk still has to be released to the baby. The involuntary reflex that forces the milk down the milk ducts is called the let-down reflex.

It usually is stimulated by the sensation of the baby's mouth on the nipple, which sends an impulse up the nerves to the pituitary gland, which in turn releases a hormone called oxytocin into the bloodstream. This travels to the breast tissue, stimulates the muscular structures, and contracts the milk ducts, forcing the milk down into the cavities behind the nipples. Within thirty to ninety seconds the milk oozes or runs from the nipples, or may even jet out in a spray for some twelve inches!

Sometimes the reason breasts become sore is because the let-down reflex is not working efficiently so milk is not being released promptly. The baby starts to chew too much, trying to get milk. Helpful hints: A relaxed attitude helps the let-down reflex happen; a warm shower or hot towels placed over the breasts can help. Also helpful is hand-expressing your milk for a few seconds before the baby nurses so that the milk is ready at your nipples when the baby starts to suck.

The handy dandy booze and snooze method.

Dr. E. Robbins Kimball, an Illinois pediatrician, the person, in fact, who started the Evanston Hospital breast milk bank, has advocated a "booze and snooze" method for nursing mothers that we have found works wonders. He describes it this way.

"Say the baby wakes crying hard. The mother changes his diapers. Still he cries. She nurses him, but the crying continues. Apparently she isn't relaxing enough to let the milk down or the baby is too upset to nurse properly.

"The father can help calm and happiness to return. He does this by settling his wife comfortably in bed or a lounge chair with the baby, then pouring her a glass of wine, mixing her a light highball or cocktail, or perhaps best of all, because of its food value, getting her a cold glass of beer. He gives her the drink and takes the baby. She drinks it, drifts off into a refreshing nap, and awakes a short time later ready to nurse her baby (research shows the baby does not get any significant alcohol in the milk from such light imbibing)."

Or, if you are a teetotaler, says Dr. Kimball, substitute hot tea for the alcohol. It's the relaxation that counts.

How do I know if my baby is getting enough to eat?

Believe us, in the not too distant future, you will be wondering how to get him to stop eating so much.

As long as your baby is not waking up at short intervals screaming and fussing, as long as it isn't losing weight, you can be pretty sure the baby is getting enough milk.

A really hungry baby does not sleep for more than an hour or so. It awakens because of hunger pangs and cries bitterly. If your baby sleeps for three or four hours after a feeding you can be fairly certain it is getting enough to eat. If it cries a lot, feed it more often and for a longer time.

At any one feeding you will soon learn to know when it is truly finished. It will relax it's clenched fists, or may produce what passes for a smile, or may simply stop sucking and contentedly fall asleep.

Remember that all babies are different and will behave

differently at the breast. Some suck and eat immediately with gusto and vigor. Others play around before seriously starting to nurse. These babies can become furious and start to scream if hurried. Others nurse awhile, rest, then start up again. You will soon learn your baby's pattern.

At about ten to fourteen days of age many babies act dissatisfied with the breast, especially during the afternoon and evening. Thus begins what may be called the "hungry age," a period of about ten days when baby develops an enormous appetite. Mothers who do not understand what is taking place often stop nursing during this time, thinking their supply of milk is diminishing. Actually the baby is increasing its demand for milk, and you simply need to nurse more frequently. The milk supply will increase to meet the baby's demands, and the baby will soon be satisfied again. This period of increased hunger and growth accompanied by a need for extra nursing often occurs again at six weeks and three months.

Your diet during breast-feeding.

A normal, high-nutrition diet is perfectly adequate for nursing. Get plenty of proteins and fresh fruits and salads just as you always should. Continue to take your prenatal daily vitamin pills, and follow the other diet advice in Chapter 12.

You should concentrate on getting plenty of fluids. See that you drink at least three quarts—that's twelve glasses of water, juice, or other fluids during each day.

Drinking milk is really not important in our well-fed society. While it is a good source of protein, protein is easily available via many other foods, such as meats and fish.

As long as you drink plenty of water, your breasts will manufacture milk for the baby. The breast glands will add the necessary protein, sugar, calcium, and other minerals. You may have an alcoholic beverage whenever you wish.

Continue to eat the same well-balanced diet as was prescribed during pregnancy. Your doctor may suggest that you eat extra protein foods, especially extra dairy products. Some mothers find that excess sweets or too many fruits may cause their babies to have diarrhea. Avoid any foods that cause you or your baby distress. You may continue to season your food however you like it.

Don't use too many stimulants. The chemicals you take in often appear in your milk. One woman we know could not understand why her baby cried and cried, wouldn't sleep, was nervous and irritable. Was it not getting enough milk, was it seriously ill, did it have colic? The more agitated the baby became, the more nervous the mother became, pouring in cup after cup of coffee to try to keep together through the harrowing experience, the days after days of turmoil. Then it dawned on her—the baby was getting the results of all her coffee drinking—he had coffee nerves at the age of three weeks!

You should also know that sometimes if you drink too much orange juice, it will produce colic in the baby.

Is there ever any reason for not nursing?

There are only a few situations in which a woman should not nurse her baby.

She should not nurse if she has tuberculosis or some other highly communicable disease.

If your breasts get very sore, or if you have a fever, call your doctor. You may have an infection that needs antibiotic treatment.

But you can safely feed from an infected breast. Nursing from an infected breast helps the affected breast glands to drain and heal much as the drainage of an abscess speeds healing.

The organisms or germs that cause most breast infections are not pathogenic to the normal baby's intestinal tract.

If there is any doubt as to the germs responsible for a breast infection, the doctor may suggest that you use a breast pump to empty the inflamed breast and feed only from the other breast until the infection has subsided.

If you are taking medicines.

Most drugs taken by a mother will be excreted in her milk, so if you are nursing, you should never take any medicines unless your doctor knows about it. With some medicines, the dangers to the baby are so great that the mother taking the medicine must stop breast-feeding.

For example, if a nursing mother is taking an anticoagulant, major life-threatening hemorrhages can occur in the baby. If the mother is receiving antibiotics, enough can go into the milk to build up allergy to antibiotics in the baby that he might have for the rest of his life.

Some laxatives taken by the mother can give a baby diarrhea. Sleeping pills can affect the baby. Aspirin, too, is passed on in milk, but in small amounts need not be a concern.

Even narcotics are passed on. If the mother takes codeine, heroin, or morphine, the nursing baby will become seriously addicted and will have the same kind of frightening withdrawal symptoms as an adult when taken off the narcotic. Marijuana also will be excreted in breast milk.

Most tranquilizers are also excreted in breast milk and they too can be addictive to the baby.

When should I wean my baby?

The time of weaning can depend on what seems best for you and your baby. You will probably want to discuss the subject with your pediatrician, who can be helpful in guiding you through this transition period.

Occasionally, weaning will be brought on involuntarily by something like flu or food poisoning that causes vomiting and diarrhea and dries you up almost overnight. But usually you are in control of the situation and can gradually wean your baby when you wish. Drop one breast-feeding every day for a week, then drop another one, substituting a bottle for those feedings. Gradually give up more and more feedings on the breast. Depending on when you wean the baby, you can switch the baby to a bottle or immediately wean the baby to a glass.

Human milk is sufficient nourishment for a baby until about age four to five months. Then the baby should have solid foods in addition to having your milk.

If you start to wean at about six months or afterwards, you can substitute a cup of milk for the feeding you drop each week. This convenient weaning to a cup enables you to skip the inconvenience of bottles totally. This also enables you to separate the association of security to food. As long as the baby suckles to get food, the two concepts are interrelated. With milk coming from a cup, the baby's security remains tied to its relationship with the mother and does not transfer to a bottle.

Supplementary bottles.

It's a good idea right from the beginning to give the baby a bottle to substitute for one nursing period. This gets baby used to accepting prepared formula from a bottle as well as milk from your breast. Then if anything should happen to you—a trip out of town, an accident or illness sending you to the hospital, whatever, your baby would not be frantic at being offered a bottle. It would already be accustomed to it.

This also gives you an opportunity to get away from the house at any time so that you can go to a movie or visit friends and have the baby-sitter give a bottle to the baby.

You may also be giving it in the hospital a bottle of dilute sugar water between feedings. To prepare dilute sugar water, add a half-teaspoon of table sugar to four ounces of boiled water. Let the baby have some whenever it is fussy between feedings, especially in hot weather, but don't give it to it just before feedings.

If you must be away from your baby for a few days, you can still resume breast-feeding on your return home. Simply take a hand breast pump with you. This is essentially a rubber bulb attached to a glass funnel to apply suction to the breast. If you use this for two minutes on each breast four times a day, the milk will continue to flow. At most it will take you and your baby one to two days on your return to fall again into the regular breast-feeding routine.

Drugs to dry up the milk supply.

It is far better to deal with natural phenomena in a natural way. Weaning as we have outlined it here goes gently and smoothly. It is possible to prescribe estrogen to speed the process of breast involution, but the use of estrogen in this regard is associated with some increased risk of deep vein clotting.

If you will be taking birth control pills, the slight amount of estrogen that they contain will help in reducing your milk supply when coupled with a weaning program.

If you do not plan to nurse, there is a hormone that can be given as a pill or an injection after delivery to help lessen engorgement. A particularly good one is pyridopine, which was found in one study to stop lactation in 95 percent of patients within one week. It suppresses painful engorgement within ten to twelve hours.

Incidentally, if after taking it you decide to nurse, it is still quite possible to do so. It merely requires extra persistence to keep the milk flowing during the first two postpartum weeks.

11

Getting That Beautiful, Svelte Figure Back

After you have your baby, you're going to walk out of the hospital tall, erect, smiling, and with a firm, flat tummy again. Right? Wrong!!

Probably one of the biggest disappointments, and one that is totally unexpected, is the discovery that your tummy isn't flat at all. You're not protruding as much as when you went into the hospital, but you're certainly protruding a lot more than you had in mind for your homeward trip. And chances are you may even have to wear your maternity outfit home because you can't get into anything skinnier.

But be of good cheer. Time and a routine of proper exercises will bring you back to the way you were.

This chapter will summarize for you the proper steps for getting back into shape again.

How soon can I expect to get back into shape?

The muscles of the abdominal wall more than double in length during the nine months of pregnancy. By the end of the fourth postpartum week they are only 10 percent longer than before pregnancy. Then, with a lot of exercise, with the passage of the next month, they reach to within 5 percent of their original length.

They almost never do better than that. This means that you usually have to give up one inch in your waistline when you have a baby. Fortunately, you only add that inch once, not with every baby.

Is there any way I can get my original waistline back?

You can unless you were in perfect physical trim before your pregnancy started. If you were an athletic sportswoman with a firm abdomen, you must give up one inch. But most women are not in peak muscular trim, so that if they exercise extensively they can probably reach their old waist measurement.

What about general exercise?

Exercise is good, and it is one of the quickest ways to get your body back to its old self again. Even in the hospital now the philosophy is that the sooner you get up and move around the better. Unless you have had major surgery during delivery, such as a cesarean, or unless you are heavily drugged or dizzy, you should get up right from the beginning to go to the bathroom. The nurse should steady you for the first walk whether or not you feel wobbly. If you feel dizzy, tell her, so that you don't faint and hurt yourself.

Every day in the hospital, get up and walk around. Walk down to the nursery and see your baby through the window, take a stroll through the halls to a lounge room if there is one, and walk your visitors to the elevator.

At home, don't do any housework for the first week. Let your husband or hired help take care of the laundry, dishes, and shopping. Play with the baby, feed the baby, and entertain your visitors.

It is quite all right to go out that first week, but someone should be with you. It is not unusual to have feelings of weakness and faintness that first week out of the hospital. For that reason you should not drive a car then.

After the first week at home you can begin to venture out alone and reaffirm your independence. Don't run or jog, but walk slowly. You can drive the car but don't act as chauffeur for arduous trips.

Stairs are safe, providing you go up and down slowly, holding on to the banister or to a companion for the first week or two. You should not bound up and down the stairs until after your postpartum checkup.

How soon after I get home can I start doing exercises?

During the first four postpartum weeks the abdominal muscles are undergoing natural involution, that is, shrinking back to their original lengths. Abdominal exercises are of no value during this time. You can firm and strengthen a muscle by voluntarily flexing it between two fixed points or by offering resistance at one movable point. The postpartum abdomen allows neither of these conditions until significant natural shortening has taken place.

In addition, you should not do physically tiring exercises until the uterus has shrunk back to its small size. If you become physically overtired you will build up acids in your bloodstream, and the uterine muscle will tend to relax and allow excessive bleeding.

Exercise 1: Vaginal contractions.

This exercise can begin just as soon as you like, even when you are lying on the delivery table if you wish. But please wait until your obstetrician has completed suturing your episiotomy so that he will not have a moving target.

The exercise consists of contracting the pubococcygeus and bulbocavernosus muscles. These are the muscles of the pelvic floor and urogenital triangle. You may have been taught to do this in your preparation-for-childbirth classes. It should be started in the hospital and should be continued at home until your postpartum checkup at four to six weeks.

Purpose: To rebuild muscle tone in the vagina, and to get the muscles that were stretched during delivery taut again. The vaginal contractions also increase circulation and drainage of the vaginal area and so help prevent infection and speed up healing. The contraction exercises improve urinary control. And they are the best thing in the world to prevent the decreased interest in sex that sometimes occurs after childbirth.

Exercise: Lie on your back with your knees in the air bent at right angles and apart. (After you get used to the exercise, you can do it sitting, standing, or in any position.) Tighten your muscles as though you were holding back urine and a bowel movement both. Do this slowly to the count of one, tighten more at two, even tighter at three, and relax to the count of four and five.

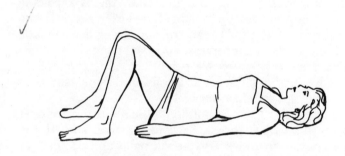

Do this a few times the first day or so while you are in the hospital. Increase the number you do, until by the time you come home you should be able to do twenty-five or fifty at a time every few hours. Try to work up to two hundred contractions total per day if you can.

When you go to the bathroom, you can test how much control you are achieving by doing the exercise to hold back your urine in spurts. Sit on the toilet with your knees apart. Start the flow of urine and then, without bringing your knees together, try to stop the flow by contracting your muscles. If your muscles are weak you will not have much control, but by the time you have done the exercises for a few weeks you should have sufficient control to be able to urinate a teaspoon at a time.

After you have good control, practice the same contractions during intercourse and you will both have new appreciations and sensations.

Exercise 2: Foot circles.

Do this while in the hospital. After you are at home you will probably be moving around enough not to need it any more.

Purpose: To increase circulation and improve muscle tone and so help prevent cramps and varicose veins.

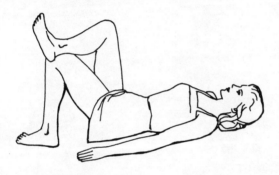

Exercise: Lie on your back in bed with your knees bent. Your feet should be flat on the bed about twelve inches from your buttocks. Rest your right ankle on the left knee. Make a large clockwise circle with your right foot. Do five times. Switch to your left foot and do five times. Then do five each in a counterclockwise direction. Try to do the entire sequence twice a day for the first week.

Exercise 3: Lactation exercise.

This may be done in the hospital beginning on day one. By the time you go home your milk supply will probably be ample enough that you can discontinue it.

Purpose: To prevent the discomfort of breast enlargement.

Exercise: Sit with your ankles crossed and feet tucked up

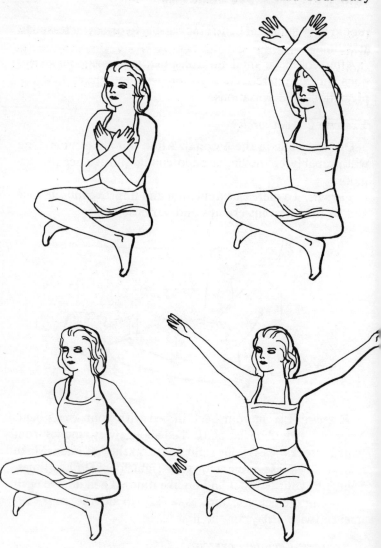

near your body, your arms resting on your lap with your wrists crossed. On count one, start to raise your arms to make large circles, starting on the inside and coming up and out. Continue up to the top of the circle on counts two and three. On counts four, five, and six, lower the arms until the fingers touch behind you as far back of the shoulders as possible, palms pointing backward. Pull arms forward quickly and place in lap again. Do five times, twice a day.

Exercise 4: The pelvic rock.

This exercise can also be done right from the start. Start doing it twice a day in the hospital and continue until your four- to six-week checkup.

Purpose: Relieves discomfort in the lower back.

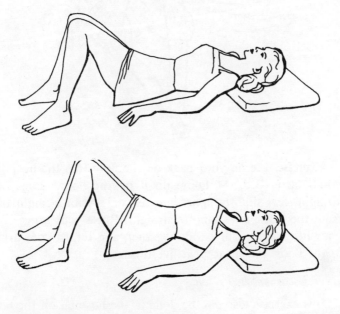

Exercise: Lie on your back with the knees and thighs together, knees bent at right angles. Soles of the feet are flat. The head can be on a pillow. Inhale slowly to the count of three. Tuck your buttocks up and flatten your lower spine against the floor at the count of four. Then return and arch your back. Repeat five times twice a day.

Exercise 5: Hand clap.

You can begin this exercise on day one or whenever you feel like it.

Purpose: To strengthen your pectoral muscles and improve circulation to the chest.

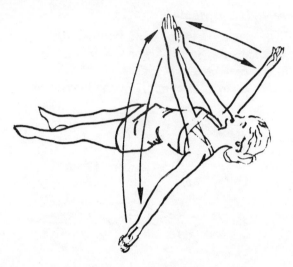

Exercise: Lie on your back on the floor. (In the hospital you'll be in bed. At home do it on the floor.) Legs out straight, feet slightly apart and relaxed. Arms straight out from the sides, with elbows straight. Raise your arms over your head, clap your hands together, and return your arms to the floor. Pause. Repeat five times.

Exercise 6: Ankle stretch.

This exercise also can be done in the hospital on the bed or at home on the floor.

Purpose: To improve muscle tone in the legs and to prevent risk of deep leg vein clotting, or thrombophlebitis, which is a risk during the postpartum period.

Exercise: Sit with your legs extended and your feet together. Your arms should be down at your side with the palms of the hands on the floor for support. Point your toes

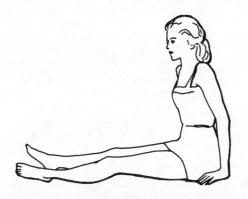

forward as far as you can. Then bend your ankles and point your toes backward toward your head.

Exercise 7: Head raising.

You can start this exercise on about day three in the hospital.

Purpose: To tighten and relax the sternomastoid muscle of the neck as an aid to neck relaxation.

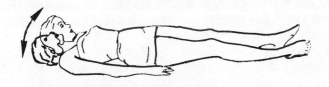

Exercise: Lie flat on your back without any pillows. Arms at your side. Raise your head and touch your chin as close to your chest as possible. Don't move any other part of your body. Repeat ten times.

Exercise 8: Upper hip roll.

This can be started a few days after the baby's birth, and can be continued indefinitely.

Purpose: To try to get your waist back to its original measurement.

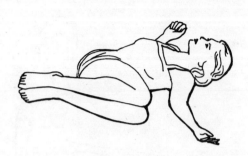

Exercise: Lie on your back. Bend your knees until they are almost up to your nose, keeping the knees together. Spread your arms out at shoulder level, with palms up. Keep both shoulders touching the bed or floor. Lower the knees to one side so knee and thigh touch the bed or floor. Return to center. Then lower knees to other side. Go back and forth from one side to the other to a slow count of three. Do it four times on each side to start. Build up gradually after you get home to ten or fifteen times or more. This is a good exercise to keep up for many years to keep your waistline in shape.

Exercise 9: Knee raise.

Don't do this exercise until after you are at home. Continue it until you start doing more strenuous exercise and feel you are no longer benefiting by it.

Purpose: To regain the normal functions of the psoas muscle whose tendon was compressed and irritated by the back

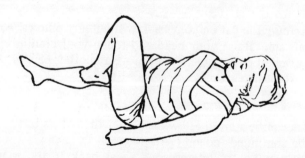

of the uterus during the last month of pregnancy.

Exercise: Lie on your back on the bed or floor. Arms comfortably at your side. Legs straight. Raise your right knee and bring it to your chest as far as possible. Lower your leg and straighten it. Alternate with right and left leg, doing each five times.

Exercise 10: Abdominal strengthening.

An exercise to start at four weeks after the baby is born.

Purpose: To strengthen the oblique muscle of the abdominal wall and get that stomach flat.

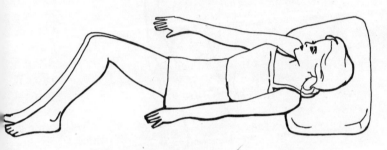

Exercise: Lie flat on your back with your head resting on a pillow. Bend your knees at a right angle, with your feet flat on the floor about twelve inches from your buttocks. Your feet, knees, and thighs are all held snugly together. Arms at the side. Raise the right arm and reach toward the left knee, but keep your left shoulder on the floor, only lifting the head and the right shoulder. Lie back. Raise the left arm and reach toward the right knee in the same way. In the beginning, hold for a count of two. By the end of a week of practice try to hold the up position for a count of five. Do at least five times on each side every day for six weeks.

Exercise 11: Torso stretch.

This can begin in the hospital or at home.

Purpose: To thin the waistline and try to return it to its former measurement.

Exercise: You can do the exercise when standing, or when lying on your back on the floor. In a standing position, look up at the ceiling and raise both arms, stretching your hands as far up toward the ceiling as you can. Feet are an inch or two apart, relaxed. Back straight with your pelvis forward. Bend your left arm slightly, at the same time stretch your right arm fully, and raise the left heel and left hip slightly. Repeat on the opposite side. Do five times each side.

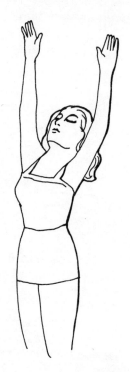

You can also do this stretch while lying on your back on the floor.

Exercise 12: Deep knee bend.

This exercise should not be done in the hospital, in fact should wait until vaginal bleeding is almost completely finished.

Purpose: To reestablish muscle tone in the leg muscles and to strengthen and spare your back.

Exercise: Stand with your feet close together. Use a chair at first for support. Later, as you build up strength, you can eliminate the chair. With one hand on the chair back (or resting on a wall) bend your knees until you are squatting, all the time keeping your knees pointed straight ahead. Then stand, keeping your back straight with your hips in line straight under your shoulders. Do not bend forward. Do not stick your hips out behind. Do only two or three of these at one time at first. Later you can do them five times, at least twice a day.

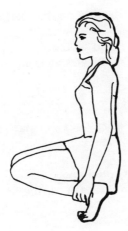

You can also put this exercise into effect when you need to open a bottom drawer, tie a shoelace, or pick something up from the floor. Simply put one foot slightly in front of the other for better balance. Picking things up this way, especially heavy weights, will prevent back sprains, strains, and pains.

Exercise 13: Pelvic elevation.

This exercise can be done after you return home, on about the tenth day.

Purpose: To strengthen the vaginal muscles and the back muscles.

Exercise: Lie on the floor on your back. Spread your legs slightly and slide your feet back toward you so that your knees are bent at almost right angles. Raise your buttocks so

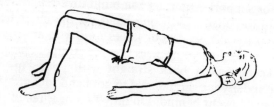

that your weight rests only on the soles of the feet and your shoulders, with your back straight. In this position, press your knees together and at the same time contract the abdominal and vaginal muscles as though you were trying to check a bowel movement.

Exercise 14: Sit-ups.

Do this exercise after your postpartum checkup. It is a good general exercise and can be continued indefinitely with good benefit.

Purpose: To flatten abdomen, and general conditioning.

Exercise: Lie on your back on the floor with your knees

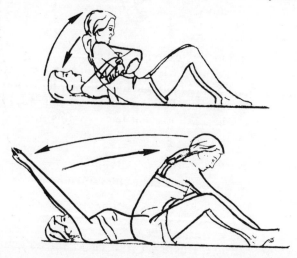

slightly elevated. Cross your arms on your chest. Raise the head and shoulders, at first just enough to clear the floor. Later, extend the arms above the head and carry through to the sitting position. Do five times to begin. Work up gradually to ten times.

Exercise 15: Pelvis rock standing.

This is an exercise for later in the postpartum period—starting in about the fourth week. It's basically the same as the pelvis rock lying down that you did earlier.

Purpose: To firm your abdomen and improve your posture.

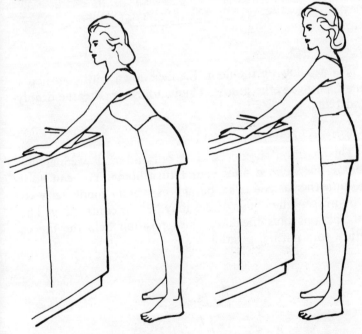

Exercise: Standing with your feet slightly apart, lift your chest, pull your stomach in, pull your shoulders back and down, pull your buttocks in, and rock your pelvis forward. Rock back to original position. Do this five times during your regular exercise time or whenever you think of it. It's good to do leaning against the sink before you do the dishes.

Prone rest.

This is a position rather than an exercise. And a welcome position too, after so many months of not being able to lie on your stomach. Remember how you used to wish fervently you could make a giant hole in your bed to stick your bulky belly in so you could lie on your stomach for a change?

The purpose of this position is to help drainage from the uterus, as well as give you a marvelous relaxing position for resting and sleeping.

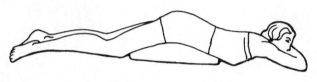

Put a pillow on the floor. Lie face down with your abdomen resting on the pillow. Thighs together. Breathe deeply and relax.

Knee–chest position.

This position should be used only after all vaginal discharge has stopped after your return home. You can do it anytime then as you relax, but it is especially good after your baby nurses when your uterus may be still contracting. The contractions plus the knee–chest position help the uterus return to a normal position.

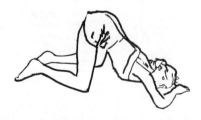

Get down on all fours. Fold your arms and place your head on them. Knees about eighteen inches apart. Back straight. This should make your derriere high in the air, with your shoulders low, so that the force of gravity is pulling your uterus into its proper position.

Take the position for about two minutes each morning and each afternoon after urinating.

If you do your knee–chest position so that your head is at the edge of your bed you can place a book or newspaper on the floor and read quite comfortably.

A good sleeping position.

One of your goals is to get back your good posture, and this means getting rid of the swayback you may have developed during pregnancy. To straighten your back and strengthen it, sleep or rest while lying on your side with one or both knees drawn up high enough to make your back flexed. You should have a firm mattress or a bed board.

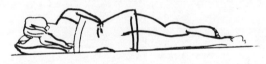

Incidentally, coming home from the hospital is a perfect time to get used to a firm mattress, since that day is very tiring and you should have no trouble sleeping.

12

Eating Your Way
Back to Best Health

The same good diet that is important to the health of the
baby during pregnancy is important to your health during
the postpartum period. It is from the building blocks of
vitamins, minerals, and proteins in your food that your body
rebuilds itself.

Poor nutrition is so easily correctable, and yet for many
new mothers who are not getting proper nutrition, life is less
than it could be as they go through day after day without
optimal health and energy.

As one physician has put it, "We pay less attention to the
care and feeding of pregnant women and new mothers than
we do to the care and feeding of our cattle, our cats, and our
dogs."

What a woman eats or fails to eat not only influences the
way she feels during the postpartum period, but also influ-

ences the speed and completeness of her recovery.

Your body is not only recovering from the stress of birth but also must recover nutritionally because any shortages of vitamins or minerals during pregnancy may have depleted your storage depots. You need to replace these reserves, as well as supply nutritive elements for healing and for rebuilding strength.

What you eat now will mean a great deal in how fast you bounce back to normal, and it will lay the foundation for solid good health for the future, both for your own vitality and for easier and safer future pregnancies and healthier babies in those future pregnancies.

This chapter will outline exactly what you need to know to eat your way back to good health.

How soon can I eat after delivery?

You can eat just as much and just as soon after delivery as you want to. Since you are not allowed to eat during labor, most women come out of the delivery room tired, but starved. In the past, new mothers would be presented with an unsavory fare of liquids and soft mush. Today mothers are given juice and a snack right away. And the next delivery of meal trays to patients will find theirs just as laden and full of food as those of the other patients. In fact, some women who have rapid labors boast that they have been able to have babies without ever missing a meal.

A very rare number of women feel nauseated for a short time after delivery, and only in these cases are diets limited to appropriate liquids or intravenous fluids, and then only until the nausea disappears.

Are any special postpartum foods given in the hospital?

You will be given lots of juices.
You will be given an ample supply of milk.
You will have protein with every meal.
You will have water at your bedside.
Take them all.
In the hospital eat whatever they give you, but eliminate the pastries if you are not pleased with your weight. This is

not a time to become up-tight, and you can trust the hospital dietician. This is also a good time to have your husband bring you some of the things you might have had to avoid in the last month or two of pregnancy—eat some pizza or marzipan candy if it makes you happy and get rid of the craving while you are in the hospital.

Are there any things you should not eat in the hospital?

You can have anything you wish, although you may have to modify your intake with experience. For example, many breast-feeding mothers report that when they eat pears, their babies soon have diarrhea.

Can I eat fruits and candy and snacks brought to me by visitors?

Yes, but you usually pay a high caloric price for the visitors' snacks.

What special diet should I have when I get home?

You should have a diet rich in protein and relatively low in fats and carbohydrates. Most women have taken on additional fat stores during pregnancy, much of this under the influence of hormones. To mobilize this fat after having the baby you should keep fats and carbohydrates to a minimum.

Decide the weight you want at the end of six weeks and calculate what your weight loss should be. It's actually rare to find anyone who doesn't want to lose weight at this time. But don't strive for a weight loss of more than a pound per week. Each day use a table of calories to calculate the calories in the food you eat. Then plan your menus.

And there is nothing wrong with saving all your calories in a day for that special restaurant you're going to in the evening.

During the first six weeks at home be sure to keep up your fluid intake, which must be three quarts a day minimum, whether you are breast-feeding or not. Make up the fluids with low-calorie fluids such as water, fruit juices, iced or warm tea, and coffee, with artificial sweeteners if necessary, and low-calorie soft drinks.

How long should I stay on this diet?

Until you are pleased with your shape.

What about alcohol or coffee?

You can take both safely. Both are excreted slightly in the milk of nursing mothers, so should not be used in excess.

Are there any vitamins and minerals that are particularly helpful to the postpartum woman?

Iron and calcium stores are usually depleted in most postpartum women. These minerals should be continued for at least two months as extra pills or as part of taking a daily vitamin pill.

The nursing mother should take calcium and iron supplements as long as she is nursing, since she will secrete these substances in her milk.

Don't go on binges.

Too much coffee can give you coffee nerves. More than two glasses of orange juice every day can give your baby colic if you nurse. More than four glasses of milk may give you too many phosphates and cause leg cramps.

A lot of licorice can give you high blood pressure.

What about wheat germ oil?

Since the 1930s there have been intermittent reports of the effects of wheat germ oil concentrate on pregnancy and its complications. It has been reported at the World Congress on Nutrition from studies on thousands of women that wheat germ oil will reduce the frequency of miscarriages, stillbirths, and premature births, and will reduce the incidence of preeclampsia and toxemia of pregnancy.

Women who took wheat germ oil during pregnancy also had slightly less postpartum bleeding and slightly shorter duration of labor.

All of the physiologic properties of wheat germ oil have not been worked out, but it is fairly clear that it does improve the ability of the body tissues to utilize oxygen and to store glycogen, which explains its value to the diet of pregnant women. However, we do not know of any studies that have been reported on taking wheat germ in the postpartum period.

But isn't the average American diet basically adequate?

No. Contrary to popular opinion, the average diet eaten by Americans is terribly inadequate. Study after study, both government and private, has come up with this same conclusion. And the bad nutrition does not occur just in poor or less educated peoples; it occurs just as often in middle class and rich groups, among the college-educated as well as dropouts. It is bad in all age groups too, with particularly bad nutrition intake found in teen-agers and the elderly.

The diet deficits are found in not just the amounts of vitamins and minerals, but also in the basic food groups.

What are the basic food groups?

The four basic food groups are: (1) the milk group; (2) the protein group of meat, fish, poultry, or eggs; (3) the vegetable and fruits group; and (4) the bread and cereal group.

The milk group includes not only whole, skim, and evaporated milk, but also butter, cheese, and ice cream. An inch cube of cheddar cheese or a cup of cottage cheese equals two-thirds cup of milk; a half cup of ice cream equals a quarter cup of milk.

The meat group includes not only meat, fish, and poultry, but also eggs, dry beans, peas, peanut butter, and nuts, because they all have necessary proteins and B vitamins.

With the high cost of eating now, a high meat diet can be a real burden on the budget. But there is no need to sacrifice nutrition for the sake of your budget with these substitutes.

For example, about the same amount of protein found in a half pound of meat can be found in: eight eggs, or eight ounces of any type of fish, or eight ounces of poultry, or one-cup dried beans or peas, or eight ounces of cheese.

Try these variations for some meals if you need to save money.

Your diet should also include four or more servings of fruits and vegetables every day, with at least one being a citrus fruit for vitamin C and another being a good source of vitamin A. Good sources of vitamin C are grapefruit, orange, cantaloupe, guava, mango, papaya, strawberries, broccoli, and green and red peppers. Foods good for vitamin A are dark green and yellow vegetables and fruits, such as apricots, broccoli, cantaloupe, carrots, collards, cress, kale, mango, pumpkin, spinach, squash, sweet potato, and turnip greens.

Breads and cereals should be those that are whole-grained.

What about between-meal snacks?

If you want them, eat them, especially if the snacks pick you up from fatigue.

Just try to make them nutritious instead of fattening. Eat proteins and salads instead of sugar and starch.

Foods for iron.

Iron deficiency is one of the most prevalent nutritional problems in women at all ages, scientists estimating some 30 million women in the U.S. right now are deficient in the essential mineral. Women particularly need iron because they lose it with blood loss during menstruation and because of added iron requirements during pregnancy.

Symptoms of iron deficiency are familiar to many of us— fatigue, weakness, pale face, heart palpitations, nail deformities, and liver disorders.

The main food sources for iron are meats (especially organ meats such as liver and kidneys), shellfish, eggs, dried beans, nuts, dark green leafy vegetables, whole-grain or enriched breads, cereals and dried fruits.

But a major problem is that all the iron in these foods is not in a form that can be absorbed by the body. Despite popular thought, for example, spinach is not a great source of iron for humans. The iron is there, but not in a form that our bodies can use. Because women seldom get enough iron naturally in foods, the Food and Drug Administration has proposed a new ruling for increasing the amount of iron added to bread and other flour products.

It's fine to eat the foods rich in iron, but to make sure that you are getting enough iron in this important period, take your iron tablets also.

What are the minimal daily requirements for vitamins and minerals?

The amounts recommended as minimum each day for an average woman are listed as follows by the U.S. Food and Drug Administration:

Calcium	1 gram
Iron	18 milligrams
Vitamin A	5000 international units
Vitamin B_1 (Thiamine)	1.5 milligrams
Vitamin B_2 (Riboflavin)	1.7 milligrams
Vitamin B_6	2 milligrams
Vitamin B_{12}	6 micrograms
Folic acid	0.4 milligrams
Niacin	20 milligrams
Vitamin C	60 milligrams
Vitamin D	400 international units
Biotin	0.30 milligrams
Pantothenic acid	10 milligrams
Phosphorus	1 gram
Iodine	150 micrograms
Magnesium	400 milligrams
Copper	2 milligrams
Zinc	15 milligrams

The new mother should be sure to get at least as many vitamins as listed for the average woman. These are *minimum* daily requirements. Many nutritionists believe the daily requirements are much higher and are trying to get these official recommended requirements increased.

The woman who is breast-feeding should get higher amounts. The following are recommended:

Calcium	1.3 grams
Iron	18 milligrams
Vitamin A	8000 international units
Vitamin B_1	1.7 milligrams
Vitamin B_2	2 milligrams
Vitamin B_6	2.5 milligrams
Vitamin B_{12}	8 micrograms

Folic acid	0.8 milligrams
Niacin	20 milligrams
Vitamin C	60 milligrams
Vitamin D	400 international units
Biotin	0.30 milligrams
Pantothenic acid	10 milligrams
Phosphorus	1.3 grams
Iodine	150 micrograms
Magnesium	450 milligrams
Copper	2 milligrams
Zinc	15 milligrams

How much weight should I lose right after delivery?

The average weight gain during pregnancy is about twenty pounds. The weight gain is divided about as follows:

Baby	7½ pounds
Placenta	1½ pounds
Amniotic fluid	1½ pounds
Increased weight of uterus	2 pounds
Stored excess fluids	6 pounds

Individuals range above and below this, of course; it is only an average.

You will lose some of the weight in delivery and during the first week in the hospital. When you return home, you will find that you weigh about fifteen pounds less than when you entered the hospital in labor. This is the time to weigh yourself and to map out your strategy.

You may find that your weight is ideal, but you don't quite look right as yet. Or you may decide that you need to lose weight and change your shape a bit. Each of these is easy to deal with.

A basic recommended postpartum weight-loss diet.

Be relaxed about food and use common sense. You can manage your diet well with a basic knowledge of calories and caloric needs, and knowing that in the postpartum period you usually have some stored extra fat that you will want to get rid of.

You need to know that fats contain nine calories per gram, protein has four calories per gram, and carbohydrates have four calories per gram. Protein has high nutritive value. So you will want to eat lots of protein and cut down as much as possible on fats and carbohydrates.

You can help figure calories by knowing a tablespoon is about fifteen grams, a teaspoon about five grams. So you can figure a tablespoon of fat contains 135 calories!

If you want to take in about fifteen hundred calories to cut your weight down, you can now plan your day.

Most nutritionists believe you need a good breakfast to give you enough energy to get through the morning. If you have two slices of toast, orange juice, an egg and coffee, that's 400 calories. If you have a glass of milk in addition, you reach 550 calories, leaving only 950 calories for the rest of the day. Try to find a happy medium that makes you most comfortable.

Keep trying to choose foods to keep protein intake high and calorie and sweet intake low.

As you work at the general principles, fit them to your own habits and preferences so that your eating will still be fun and not just a chore.

And be sure to include foods from the basic food groups to keep up your proper nutrition.

A program for losing weight.

There are many fad diets for losing weight, but the best way for sure to safely and surely lose weight is to cut down your sugars and carbohydrates and take in fewer calories than you expend in energy every day.

Here's how to figure up the number of calories you should consume in the average day.

Most people use about 15 calories per pound to maintain their weight. So if you weigh 120 pounds and you want to stay there you should take in no more than 120 × 15, that is, 1800 calories per day.

To lose a pound a week you need to reduce your calorie intake by 500 calories a day. So if you weigh more than your ideal weight, say 130, and want to lose, you can lose one pound a week by consuming 500 *fewer* calories per day. Taking in 1300 calories a day instead of 1800 would gradually bring you down to 120 pounds. Once you get there, you can resume your maintenance level of 1800 calories per day.

What if I still have a lot of fluid in my tissues?

The fluid will redistribute itself and be excreted naturally as your hormone levels fall to normal. It's not wise to take diuretics (water pills) since the natural phenomena are adequate. You can speed up the process by limiting salt in your diet. Caffeine is a diuretic and so some extra coffee will help also, as will tea.

Other tips on losing weight.

It is important that you do not go on a crash diet to lose weight because you need all the essential basic foods and vitamins and minerals to build yourself up. The way to lose weight now is by gradually cutting down high-carbohydrate and high-calorie foods, but still eating the foods that you need for energy and body building.

Here are some hints for slow and safe reducing in the postpartum period.

Purchase a small calorie-counting book and consult it in selecting foods. Choose the foods that are high in nutrition and low in calories.

Remove high-calorie foods from your diet. Eat no bread. Replace sugar with artificial sweetener. Eliminate sugary desserts. Watch out for cocktails and beers, high in calories.

Keep a ready supply of low-calorie snacks handy at all times.

Build up to an adequate amount of exercise. Take the baby for a walk if the weather is nice. Get yourself out for a walk, alone or with your husband, as often as you can. The daily exercise will not only help burn up calories, but will also improve your circulation and muscle tone. Build up to more strenuous exercise as you get the time and strength.

Set up new habit patterns concerning foods. Starting a new life is always the easiest time to initiate new habits and break old ones. How you eat is basically a habit. Use the principles of behavioral control to set up negative thoughts about the foods you want to avoid and set up enthusiastic positive attitudes toward healthful food and how the proper weight is going to make you feel so much better and more energetic.

As you set up your new behavior patterns, the new habits will soon be automatic and can establish an entire new life-style. Don't worry about occasional transgressions. It's the overall pattern you're looking for.

Other tricks:

Take a "before" photograph of yourself while pregnant or when you first start your diet, showing your bulging belly, and post it in the kitchen as a constant reminder.

Put a survival kit in the refrigerator and keep it stocked with celery, carrot sticks, oranges, radishes, low-cal soda, and other low-calorie items for snacks.

Stay out of the kitchen as much as possible. Try to feed the baby elsewhere whenever possible.

Reward yourself for good behavior. When you've lost five pounds, celebrate with flowers on the table. For ten, have candlelight and silver or a trip to the theater. For reaching your recommended weight, buy yourself a lovely gift.

What about pills for losing weight?

Most pills for losing weight are a form of amphetamines or "speed." They have numerous side effects such as changes in mood and increased nervousness and changes in blood pressure, and they cause addiction. In addition, many patients have found that they gain back the weight lost on diet pills when they stop the pills.

You can discuss this with your doctor; chances are he'll try to discourage you from using them.

What is the value of losing weight?

It increases your chances for better health and longer life.

Women who are severely overweight have three times more high blood pressure than women who are not overweight. And they have higher rates of heart attacks and strokes.

Being overweight is so detrimental to your health that

physicians at the Metropolitan Life Insurance Company say you can roughly calculate how long you will live by how fat you are. Their statistics show that policyholders who are 30 percent or more overweight have a mortality rate 35 percent higher than those policyholders who weigh less. In fact, life insurance companies for many years have charged obese individuals a higher premium because their risks of dying early are greater.

And while we are on the subject of fat, please don't try to make your baby fat. A fat baby is *not* a healthy baby. In fact, generally a fat baby and a fat child will grow up to be a fat adult. If you start him out with bad eating habits he may have them all his life.

What about cholesterol and fats?

Cholesterol is a waxy material that forms part of the fatty deposits that can plug up vital arteries to bring on heart attacks or strokes. Some scientists, but not all, believe if you eat low amounts of cholesterol, and reduce consumption of saturated or "hard" fats, it will help reduce blood cholesterol levels and fatty deposits in arteries. Long-term studies are now being carried out to see if the theory is true.

Cholesterol content is high in such foods as butter, eggs, cheese, and animal fats.

What are saturated and unsaturated fats?

Saturated fats are those that are hard at room temperature. They are found in most meat, in butter, cream, and whole milk, in some cheeses, in many solid and hydrogenated shortenings, and in coconut oil, cocoa butter, and palm oil.

Polyunsaturated fats, which are recommended, are usually liquid oils of vegetable origin—oils such as corn, cottonseed, safflower, sesame seed, soybean, and sunflower seed.

The Prudent Diet.

Several groups, including the American Heart Association, have now endorsed a diet called the Prudent Diet, which takes into account several theories about the roles diet plays in high blood pressure and heart disease. It is an excellent diet for the postpartum woman.

Principles of the Prudent Diet are these:

Reduced calories

Reduced total fat

Increased polyunsaturates

Reduced dietary cholesterol

Adjusted carbohydrates (deriving carbohydrates from grain, fruits, and vegetables instead of sugars)

Reduced salt intake

Stabilized protein intake (Protein should contribute 12 percent to 15 percent of each day's calories.)

A summary of recommended diets.

You need more than a diet to cut calories, more than a diet of girth control. You need a diet to give you all the essentials for renewal of your body and mind.

You need more than a diet to reduce cholesterol and saturated fats. You need a diet to change flabby fat to lean meat.

Here are our recommended postpartum diets to fulfill all these special needs.

In the hospital.

Drink lots of water and juice.

Eat fruit and bulk foods such as salads and leafy vegetables.

Eat protein with every meal.

The first six weeks at home.

Eat a diet high in protein.

Eat only small amounts of fats and carbohydrates.

Take iron and calcium tablets every day, as well as vitamin pills. You may continue your prenatal vitamin since it contains calcium and iron.

Drink three quarts of fluid every day.

Do not drink more than four glasses of milk per day.

Count calories to take off about one pound per week.

The first year.

Drink one or two glasses of milk or servings of milk products.

Eat meat, fish, poultry, or eggs every day.

Eat green and yellow vegetables every day.

Eat citrus fruits or juice every day.

Take supplements of vitamins and minerals if there is any doubt in your mind that you are not eating a completely balanced diet.

Maintain your ideal regular weight by reducing carbohydrates and calories when necessary and reducing fat intake.

Cut down on cholesterol and saturated hard fats.

Cut down on sugars and starches.

If you breast-feed your baby.

Do not drink more than two glasses of orange juice a day, nor more than three cups of coffee or tea, nor more than four glasses of milk.

Take iron and calcium supplements.

Don't go on binges of certain foods or drinks that can affect your baby through your milk.

If you take birth control pills.

Women on birth control pills do not absorb folic acid as readily as other women. A folic acid deficiency can cause anemia, weakness, and tiredness. To correct this, be sure your diet contains green leafy vegetables, or take a supplemental vitamin containing folic acid.

13

Getting Back to Sex

Margaret D. was a rather shy girl who had always considered herself a bit old-fashioned, and certainly not a swinging sexpot in her wildest dreams.

But she found that after she came home from the hospital she had a fantastic sexual appetite. She really wanted her husband, needed him physically as she never had before.

And, she found, the sexual feelings she shared with her husband were even deeper now than they had ever been before. They had produced a magnificent new human life together; she was not only in love with her man, she was also the mother of his child.

Some women, after having a baby, find an increase in their appreciation and enjoyment of sex, as Margaret did. Others find at first that they have less interest and enjoyment in sex.

The postpartum period is one in which you will be resolving your feelings toward yourself as a new mother. This will involve a new appraisal of your relationship with your own mother and father, with your husband, and with the real and the fantasy baby you dreamt about when you were pregnant.

As you integrate these feelings, and as you redefine yourself, your sexual interest will return, usually before your postpartum examination.

When is sex safe again?

Most doctors tell their patients not to have sex before their six-week examination. Most patients do have sex before their examination. Is there an unspoken code here? Do the patients know something the doctors don't know?

Let us analyze the pertinent changes that make sex safe again; perhaps we can suggest some rational rules. Certainly the episiotomy should be totally healed before intercourse is resumed. The episiotomy begins to heal as soon as the stitches are placed, with the edges of the skin healing by the fifth or sixth day. However, the underlying tissues require two weeks to approach their previous strength, which is not really reached until the third week.

And certainly intercourse should not be resumed nor anything placed in the vagina until danger of uterine infection has passed. The uterus is protected by the cervix and by the cervical mucus-secreting glands. The cervix must close to provide a protective chemical barrier also. The cervical changes are completed by the end of the fourth week in 95 percent of new mothers.

Therefore, you can be assured of the following:

1. Sex outside the vagina is safe after the second or third week.

2. Intercourse and intravaginal sex is safe by the end of the fourth week if your cervix is closed and secreting normal mucus.

There is only one way to know if condition two exists—that is, to have your postpartum examination at the end of the fourth week. Most doctors will readily comply with your request to have your examination at four weeks, particularly if you explain your reasons. And you and your husband should easily be able to wait until then, particularly since you now know condition number one.

What about masturbation?

Masturbation is safe at any time, providing no injury occurred to the regions of the front of the vulva during delivery. However, even in a simple, uncomplicated delivery the vulva becomes swollen, and the swelling does not subside until the fourth or fifth day.

External petting and oral sex are usually safe by the second or third week, but the uncontrolled nature of the postpartum discharge (called lochia) usually makes oral sex undesirable. It is perfectly safe to stimulate the clitoris and to have an orgasm during this period, but not to have anything in the vagina.

The reason that masturbation by the woman herself can be done earlier than stimulation by her husband is that the woman is more sensitive to what will cause pain and irritation and what will not.

What will it be like the first time?

The first intercourse must be very gentle and careful. The vagina, after the stretching processes of birth and in healing from the episiotomy, frequently becomes slightly tight. In addition, most new mothers are slightly wary at this time and tend to tighten the vagina further, either consciously or unconsciously.

Realizing this, you should procede slowly, relying on manual stimulation and petting to help to stretch the vagina. It is also helpful to use a surgical lubricant (available at any drugstore or from your doctor) to be sure that the frictional resistance of the vaginal walls is reduced.

Are there any positions that should be avoided?

Any position that is comfortable is safe, but probably the most gentle one to start with is lying face to face on your sides. The most tender parts of the vagina are the parts that are stitched, the parts toward the anus. Entry from the rear would stretch this area the most and will be uncomfortable at first. Anal intercourse should also be avoided during this time.

What to do for tightening of the vagina.

Your husband should use his fingers to gently dilate your vagina. He should first insert one finger and move it about, gently pressing the walls of the vagina. There should be adequate lubrication. He then should insert two fingers and methodically press them against all the walls of the vagina. This should be done slowly, deliberately, gently, and systematically.

Finally, he should be able to insert three fingers. When the vagina is tight, you should not hesitate to spend many sessions doing dilation, building up to three fingers before you even attempt intercourse again.

What effect does breast-feeding have on intercourse?

Women who breast-feed their children have a faster return of their sexual desire, Masters and Johnson found in their studies. They did not investigate whether or not this was a physical consequence or whether this represented a psychological difference.

But women who breast-feed are more apt to have a mechanical difficulty in initiating intercourse and in finally feeling that their vagina has returned to normal during intercourse. They may not have the "normal feeling" in some instances until after they have weaned the baby.

This occurs because while the woman is breast-feeding the pituitary gland is usually inhibited from its normal cycle. That is why the nursing mother usually does not menstruate. The pituitary gland rests and does not release FSH, the ovary-stimulating hormone. The ovary, when not stimulated, produces little or no estrogen. The vagina is one of the organs affected by estrogen, and without it the vagina frequently tightens and dries abnormally. This same change often happens in women after the menopause.

After menopause the condition is treated with estrogen, given orally or placed in the vagina as a cream or ointment. Oral estrogen early in the postpartum period will usually diminish the flow of milk in the nursing mother, so she should use local estrogen. If you tell your doctor that your vagina feels tight he can prescribe an estrogen cream that you can insert into your vagina with your finger or with an applicator. Later, in about your third month, you can take low doses of estrogen without reducing your milk supply. A convenient way to do this is by using low-dosage birth control pills.

If you and your husband have sexual difficulties.

According to Masters and Johnson, more than half of the married couples in the United States suffer some kind of sexual dysfunction. It may be impotence, premature ejaculation, difficulty in having an orgasm, or discomfort with intercourse.

Causes can be simple or complex. Cures can be as simple as using a lubricant jelly, as interesting as having the woman take testosterone (male hormone) pills to increase the size of the clitoris and increase libido, or as straightforward as correcting an iron deficiency that might be causing excessive fatigue. Some people have even solved their problems by watching pornographic films together. Sexual hang-ups can be due to lack of basic communication in all aspects of a marriage or they can be due to a partner's lack of proper personal hygiene. Sitting down and talking about it, telling each other what you really like best, what turns you on—or off—can make a world of difference, not just sexually, but also in opening up new avenues of communication that did not exist before. Sometimes psychotherapy or hypnosis is beneficial.

Talk over the problem with your gynecologist. Don't be embarrassed, whatever the problem. No matter what you say, he's heard it before. You can analyze the problem together and come up with some approaches to try.

If these approaches don't produce a solution for you, you may want to consider some of the sex clinics that have been established in all parts of the country modeled after the one first established by Masters and Johnson in St. Louis. These clinics apply both psychological and physical factors in order to solve problems and they have helped thousands of couples.

Be sure the clinic counselors have had at least a year's training in an established clinic. Check with your doctor to be sure.

The big flap about vaginal sprays.

Doctors are seeing more irritations of the vaginal area now than they have ever seen before. Reason?—the increased use of feminine deodorant sprays, colored and perfumed toilet paper, and some detergents. If you have mild burning or irritation of the vaginal area, one of these might well be the cause. If the burning or irritation is severe, it could be something more serious like venereal disease, and you should immediately contact your doctor.

Despite television commercials to the contrary, there is no evidence that vaginal sprays will combat vaginal odor any better than plain soap and water. In fact, the Federal Food and Drug Administration has requested that manufacturers of the sprays be banned from using the words "hygiene" or "hygienic" on the product or its advertising.

"The FDA knows of no medicinal or hygienic benefits derived from these sprays," the agency said in announcing the ban.

Vaginal sprays can cause problems and should carry labels warning women of their dangers, according to the Food and Drug Administration. Reports have come in from hundreds of women with complaints of infections, itching, burning irritation, vaginal discharge, rashes, and other problems from the sprays.

In fact, the FDA proposes that a warning label should be put on all vaginal sprays that says, "Caution—for external use only. Spray at least eight inches from skin. Use sparingly and not more than once daily to avoid irritation. Do not use this product with a sanitary napkin. Do not apply to broken, irritated, or itching skin."

If you use a vaginal spray, you should consult a physician if a rash or irritation or discharge occurs, or if an unusual odor develops.

To douche or not to douche.

There is no reason for modern women to douche. The vagina for the most part is a self-cleansing organ. The glands of the cervix secrete a mucous substance that slowly runs out of the vagina carrying with it trapped debris and germs. Merely wiping the lips of the vagina is then sufficient to cleanse the cavity.

If you would like to clean it further, you can put your finger into the vagina during your shower or bath and enable water to enter. You can even put a little soap on your finger to help loosen any dried material, but you should be sure not to leave any soapy residue.

What to do if you have a vaginal discharge different from normal.

This is one time that a douche is useful. Using a comfortably warm solution of salt water once a day for a few days will usually clear up most mild infections.

But even here, you don't need to douche if you prefer not to. If you add half a cup of table salt to a bathtub of water you will have a good approximation of physiological saline, or normal body fluid. This would be similar to your tears, which are constantly forming and bathing your eyes. If you sit in this salty bath you can put your finger into your vagina and enable the salty water to enter. Moving your finger about will wash out the excess discharge. This is an excellent first line of attack against most vaginal infections.

The saline bath will reduce the population of any invading or excessive organisms and enable your own body defense mechanism to do a better job in fighting the infection. Nine out of ten times a few of these baths at bedtime will clear up the infection and save a trip to the doctor's office.

What is trichomoniasis?

Trichomoniasis is an infection of the body caused by trichomonas vaginalis, a vaginal parasite. It looks much like the amoeba you once saw under a microscope and it is about the same size—that is, microscopic.

It rarely causes any damage, but it does cause a smelly vaginal discharge and itching.

"Trich" is an infection of the intestinal tract also; and it is carried by the man, even though he may have no symptoms. Therefore, you must be treated with an orally administered medicine that will go through your entire system, or else the infection will come back. A vaginal medicine is not enough because recontamination of the vagina from the anus is very easy.

And your husband must be treated also, or else he will recontaminate you the next time you have intercourse.

What is moniliasis?

Moniliasis, a fungus infection, also called candidiasis, is an infection that arises from within the vagina itself. It is not spread by sexual activity.

The vagina has normal germs within it. These are called vaginal flora and, with the vaginal secretions, make up the ecology of the vagina. Part of the flora of the vagina are the monilia, or yeast cells. They live on the sugar content of the vaginal secretions.

Moniliasis is the vaginal condition that occurs when the yeast cells of the vagina multiply excessively. This results in a white discharge with curdlike particles resembling cottage cheese. It usually itches greatly, and you probably remember scratching your vulva in your sleep if you have had it. Gynecologists at a conference on common gynecological problems agreed that most women get it a few times a year. They usually learn to treat it themselves since the itching is so characteristic. It is treated by using an intravaginal antifungus agent in pill or cream form, but it also usually subsides after a few saline baths. The salty bath washes out the excess population of fungus cells and also reduces the sugar content of the vagina, so that the fungus cannot multiply as rapidly.

Moniliasis occurs whenever the ecology of the vagina is disturbed. For example, if you are given systemic antibiotics for an infection elsewhere in your body, the antibiotics might also kill off the normal germs of your vagina, allowing the fungus cells to overgrow unopposed.

Or, if the sugar content of your vaginal secretions increases, the fungus will have increased nourishment, and will multiply and cause infection. This can occur under influence of the hormones of pregnancy, or sometimes from birth control pills, or if there is too much sugar in your diet, or in diabetes. It can also occur at times of emotional stress and depression since the vaginal ecology is changed then too.

14

The Postpartum Checkup

Frances G. was ordinarily a warm, loving, outgoing person who enjoyed life. After she had her baby, she could barely drag herself around the house. She was tired and listless, even had trouble getting the diapers laundered and the formula made each day. By evening she was too tired to do the dishes and she had no interest whatsoever in making love with her husband, even though they had not been together for more than two months. Her whole life seemed to be falling apart.

When she went in for her postpartum checkup almost in tears she told her doctor what was happening. Her problem, he said, was common, and there could be a number of factors involved, both physical and psychological. So first he suggested they do the complete examination to check for any physical problems. In Frances's case a low blood count turned out to be the problem. She had simple iron deficiency anemia. Her doctor prescribed iron pills to be taken between meals every day, and within ten days she was beginning to feel more like her old self.

This is the typical problem solving that happens at the postpartum checkup.

The checkup gives you a chance to gather yourself together physically and emotionally and to examine and talk over your adjustment as a new mother.

It gives the physician a chance to check you out physically —to make sure your stitches have healed properly, your uterus has returned to normal size and position, and no complications have occurred that need treatment. This gives you the reassurance that your body is returning to normal again.

It gives you a chance to ask any questions you may have, either about physical problems or about any problems of coping and adjustment in your new life.

It also gives you a chance to discuss future sex relations and any future pregnancies, and obtain advice about them.

When should I have the postpartum exam?

The time of the examination varies from doctor to doctor. Some doctors see their patients as early as three weeks after delivery, and others as late as six to eight weeks. And often, this is individualized by choosing a time appropriate to the type of delivery and to the emotional needs of the patient.

You can certainly express your preference at the time of your discharge from the hospital. If you feel that you would rather be seen earlier, tell your doctor. It might be because you feel insecure, perhaps just to enable an earlier trip to the Caribbean to swim. The doctor will cooperate.

Should I ever see my doctor before that?

Only if you have some special problem.

You should call him, for example, if you have chills or fever, increased vaginal bleeding, severe pains in the chest or abdomen or legs, bleeding nipples or tenderness, inflammation or lumps in the breasts.

What will the postpartum examination consist of?

Your doctor will talk to you about any special problems you might be having, psychologically or physically.

He will give you a thorough physical examination, including examination of your abdominal wall and your ovaries, uterus, and vagina to see what changes have occurred, if everything is returning properly to normal, or if there are any irregularities to be corrected. He will check on how well your episiotomy has healed and whether your uterus has returned to prepregnancy size and proper location. He will check your cervix for any inflammation. If there is inflammation, irritation, or excessive mucus, he may prescribe treatment. He will inspect your breasts, checking your nipples and your breast tissue.

If it is due, he will do a Pap (Papanicolaou) smear for cancer, and also a vaginal-cell smear to determine if your estrogen is at a normal level.

He will check your blood pressure. (A good blood pressure is 120/80.) If you were anemic on discharge from the hospital, he will check your blood counts and hemoglobin level. (Normal hemoglobin is about 14 grams-percent.)

You will also spend some time talking together about your future diet and exercise programs, what your diet supplements should be, what your plans are for any future children, and the kind of birth control methods you will be using.

If you will be using birth control pills, he will instruct you in how to take them. They can usually be started at this time, unless you are nursing.

If you are going to use an intrauterine device, he will insert it at this time if he finds that your uterus has involuted sufficiently. If he finds that it is not yet back to normal, he will tell you when to return.

Usually he will wait until after you have resumed your normal sexual life before fitting a diaphragm. Or it might be fitted at the postpartum examination and you may have to return to check the fit.

What if I feel perfectly all right—can I skip the postpartum exam?

Too many things can be amiss at this time, even if you are feeling perfect.

An ovarian cyst might have grown behind the uterus during your pregnancy; this is the first time it can be discovered.

Your uterus may not be sufficiently involuted; without medicine to keep it contracting, you might be in danger of bleeding excessively. Or your cervix may not have closed sufficiently so that sexual intercourse could cause an infection.

A breast lump may be present that could not be found during the relative engorgement of the breasts during the last few months of pregnancy.

This is a small sampling of why you must come for your examination no matter how well you feel.

When should I see my doctor again?

Your next visit will depend very much on what was found during the postpartum examination. If your examination was normal, as it usually is, the timing of a return visit will in great measure depend on what you are doing for birth control and on when your next Pap smear is due.

At the very least, you must have a Pap smear and be examined gynecologically once a year until you are thirty-five years old. After that you should be examined every six months, with the Pap smear once a year.

You are responsible for preserving your own health. It is all very well to be existential about certain matters, that is to say, "what happens, happens; it is out of my control." But that philosophy does not apply in a gynecologic sense. For the most part, all the cancers that gynecologists find in their patients are curable if the patient will just allow the gynecologist to examine her twice a year and to do the Pap smear yearly, and if she will examine her own breasts monthly and report danger signals.

Why is the Pap smear so important?

The "Pap" test was developed by Drs. G. H. Papanicolaou and H. F. Traut in 1943 using cast-off epithelial (surface) cells from the cervix that are normally found in secretions obtained from the cervix. They are stained and viewed under the microscope where any malignant or premalignant cells present are seen as cells with large nuclei.

Only about 15 percent of U.S. women have had the smear

for cervical cancer—which with cancer of the breast is one of the major cancer hazards to women.

A Pap smear can predict cervical cancer before it has occurred, in its earliest stages, when it is always curable. It can show premalignant changes of the cervix, in fact, before cancer has even developed, with slight abnormalities of cells of the surface tissue in the cervix being detected.

At early stages, and even at the advanced state when the surface of the cervix has become 100 percent abnormal, most women have no symptoms. Many still have no symptoms even when the disease has progressed to invasive carcinoma that has developed and spread beyond the cervix to other tissues.

If the smear reveals unusual patterns of cells, then further tests are done. If a beginning cancer seems likely, then treatment can be started immediately.

In general, the standard treatment for women who have already had their families or have passed thirty-five years of age would be hysterectomy (surgical removal of the uterus).

In a young woman anxious to have a family, local treatment might be used—either local excision, cryosurgery, or extensive cauterization. The patient may then go ahead and have the family that she wants without much danger, providing that she is followed carefully with repeated Pap smears.

Self-examination of the breasts.

You should know how to perform self-examination of your breasts. If you do not, your doctor or his nurse can show you how at your postpartum checkup.

You should examine your breasts every month by this method, as a way of looking out for breast cancer. An astounding 90 percent of breast cancers are discovered by women themselves! And as with any cancer, the earlier the detection and treatment, the better the chances. When breast cancer is discovered in an early stage, there is an 85- to 90-percent cure rate. Once it has spread to the lymph nodes, the survival rate drops to 50 percent. So it is essential to contact your doctor immediately, if you note any abnormality.

If you discover it early enough, the treatment can be very

simple—merely removing the lump cures it.

When you examine yourself, you should check to see if there is any change in shape or size of either breast and whether there are any lumps, depressions, puckering of the skin, or unusual discharge from the nipples.

Many times when you stop breast-feeding, the breasts will have a lumpy feel to them. Don't panic.

These are merely glands that still have milk in them, and the body has not yet absorbed the milk. Wait about a month after you have stopped breast-feeding to evaluate your breasts.

How to do it.

Choose the same time each menstrual cycle, about one week after your period has started.

Stand as straight as you can, and place your arm alongside your head, against your ear, with your forearm folded across the top of your head. This maneuver stretches the breast of that side against your chest wall.

Hold your opposite hand straight with fingers together and feel your breast by pressing your palm against the breast, compressing it against your ribs and chest wall. It's important not to feel with your fingers, but rather with your palm. Your fingers would feel the irregularities of the breast glands, and that can be confusing. But your palm will only feel either a smooth feeling, or a nodule which should be reported to your doctor.

A tumor or cyst will feel like a peanut or a pea or a lima bean inserted into your breast.

Repeat the process for the opposite side.

What are other abnormal signs I should look for?

Occasional irregularities in the nature of your period or occasional extra bleeding during the month can occur in all normal women. You should report any abnormality that has occurred for more than one cycle.

Any bleeding whatsoever after the menopause should be reported to your gynecologist.

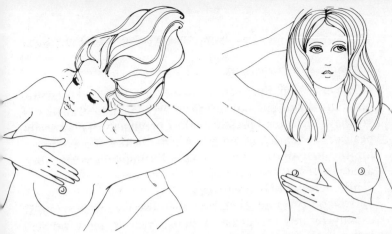

Figure A—Gently feel for a lump or thickening of the breast while you bathe or shower; lie down with one hand behind your head. With the other hand, fingers flattened, gently feel the opposite breast, pressing very, very lightly. Repeat with the other breast.

Figure B—The same procedure (gently feeling all parts of each breast) is repeated while you stand with your hand behind your head.

Figure C—Beginning at the "A" in the drawing, and following the direction indicated by the arrows, feel all parts of each breast for a lump or thickening.

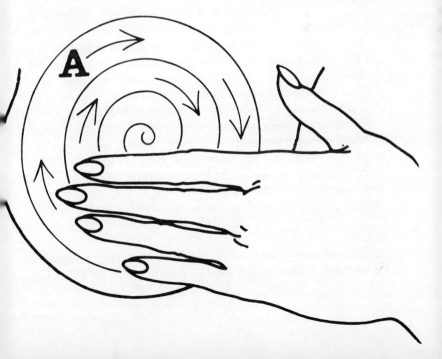

Postpartum hypertension.

Hypertension, the scientific name for high blood pressure, occurs in about one out of fifteen pregnancies. Strangely, if you have high blood pressure before pregnancy, it may disappear, or conversely, if you never had it before, it may appear for the first time. It may appear during pregnancy, then disappear. Or it may be normal during pregnancy and suddenly increase after pregnancy.

If blood pressure is high at the postpartum checkup, it usually returns to normal within a year in most women. However, some doctors consider postpartum hypertension an early sign of latent high blood pressure and urge that such women keep a regular watch on their blood pressure, obtaining treatment if their diastolic (lower) number is consistently higher than ninety-five.

High blood pressure can be dangerous, causing heart failure, strokes, kidney disease, and even death, so every woman should have her blood pressure checked during pregnancy and after delivery. In fact, everyone should have his blood pressure checked at least once a year.

Must the doctor always have a nurse present at the examination?

Some doctors still routinely have an assistant present for all pelvic examinations, but in general the old tradition has been outgrown. The nurse may or may not be there.

The American College of Obstetricians and Gynecologists has no special rulings or policy one way or the other.

Most women are more at ease if fewer eyes are around while they are being examined. If you have a special preference, you can tell your gynecologist. If he is used to working alone in the examining room he may have a buzzer to use to summon his assistant.

Have the women's liberation movement and self-help clinics made any difference in postpartum exams?

We certainly hope so. The main feature of the movements is to make women more aware of themselves, their bodies, and their rights. This can only help communication between patients and their doctors.

It is your responsibility to point out what you consider faults in your doctor or his treatment, or problems in understanding your doctor, just as it is his responsibility to ask you to repeat or explain something that he does not understand.

There are two sorts of continuing medical education for the doctor. One is what he continues to learn by attending seminars and meetings and by reading books and journals. The other is what he learns from his patients as time goes on what their real needs and problems are. And it's your job to communicate these to him.

You don't need dramatic ploys, like flinging off the sheets, to do the job. Straightforward discussion and questioning will increase your knowledge and your gynecologist's understanding of what your needs and his responsibilities are.

What can women do to take more active responsibility for their own bodies?

It is a woman's responsibility to know her anatomy, including the necessary vocabulary to describe her organs and functions. Certainly your doctor should fill you in on any terms or physiology that you don't know, but you should not expect him to give you your basic biology course.

Betty Friedan has expressed a woman's role in regard to health care succinctly. She has stated, "Doctors have been getting away with murder. The passivity of women has made it possible for doctors to treat them in an authoritative way, as if they were children." It's certainly wrong for a doctor to treat you condescendingly, but it is just as wrong for you to be passive and poorly prepared as a woman.

Can a woman really do her own pelvic examination and pregnancy tests and other things usually done by a gynecologist?

The mechanics of a pelvic examination are easy and can be mastered readily by the amateur. But the gynecologist, because of his training and experience, is much more sensitive to the nuances of subtle changes in a patient's history or physical examination, and to their relevance in health or in the progress of illness.

So we do not recommend substituting do-it-yourself examinations for regular checkups with the gynecologist. It is only by going to your doctor regularly that you will know that you are completely healthy and will be able to catch any problems in their early stages when they can be most effectively treated.

15

Family Planning
for the Future

When you have your postpartum examination you will have
the opportunity to discuss with your doctor what your op-
tions are as to methods of birth control. The social, ethical,
economical, and psychological reasons for using birth control will vary from person to person. But the medical reasons
for spacing pregnancies are applicable to everyone.

There are important physical reasons for spacing your
children. Planned spacing gives your body a chance to regain
its strength and return to a normal state.

It takes about three months for your muscles to involute,
and your body stores of vitamins and important minerals
such as iron and calcium may not become normal until after
six months or more. So that no matter how you feel about
birth control socially or philosophically, you should for
health reasons not immediately become pregnant again. Un-

less you are going to abstain completely from intercourse, you should be prepared to make an appropriate choice of birth control and use it for at least six months. After that time you can decide whether you wish to continue or to become pregnant again.

In this chapter we will tell you about all the available methods and the statistics on how effective they are, and give you the information you need to choose the method that will fit your habits and personality and goals.

Why one out of three women fail with their contraceptives.

The unbelievable statistics of one out of three failures in contraception were revealed in a national study, the results of which have recently been published by Drs. Norman Ryder and Charles Westoff, of Princeton University. Their study of a sample of almost seven thousand women showed that more than a third of the women practicing birth control over a five-year period became pregnant anyway.

In a press conference after publication of the study, Dr. Ryder said, "People have to get used to the fact that there is an awful lot of contraceptive failure in a society even as sophisticated as ours. It is nonsense to say that Americans are now having the number of children that they want."

The main reasons for contraceptive failures: use of an ineffective method, or carelessness in using a good method.

The Ryder report showed the following failure rates: Of women using a pill or intrauterine devices, 5 percent failed to prevent pregnancy in a year's time. Of couples using condoms, 10 percent failed to prevent pregnancy. Of those using diaphragms, 17 percent failed to prevent pregnancy. Of those using foams or the rhythm method, 20 percent became pregnant. Of those douching for birth control, 40 percent became pregnant during the year.

Roman Catholic women were as successful in preventing pregnancies as other women. Education levels did not seem to be a significant factor, Dr. Ryder said.

But failure rates were higher among younger women than older women, he said.

The age difference, he said, supports other findings that women who really do not want any more children are much more successful in preventing pregnancy than those who are simply trying to postpone or space their children.

"Success in contraceptive use depends in large part on the degree of motivation of the couple concerned," he said.

So the important thing—if you don't want another baby right away—is to make sure the method you use is really effective. And then, after you find the contraceptive that is best for you, be sure you use it each time and follow directions precisely and meticulously. Don't skip—even once, that's just the time you will get pregnant!

Here is a comparison of various methods.

Douching.

Forget about this as a method of birth control. It has no place in birth control nor any place as a routine measure in the life of any normal woman. Women who douche after intercourse may already be too late to prevent pregnancy. A uterine suction created during intercourse helps transport sperm upward into the uterus and fallopian tubes; the sperm thus may be streaming into the uterus within a few seconds after intercourse. Douching does nothing but give you an unnecessary, bothersome job to do.

Rhythm method.

This too is unreliable. Having intercourse only on the days before menstruation and for a few days after, and trying to guess when you are fertile to avoid that time, is dangerously unsure. You have to keep charts and calendars, which is a big bother. And if your feelings don't follow the charts, you're apt to take a chance and get caught. In addition, it has been shown that sperm can live in the fallopian tube for eleven days, just waiting for the ovum to present itself for fertilization.

To make the system even less reliable, the ovum is not always produced on schedule, but can vary from cycle to cycle.

Breast-feeding.

There is no way to predict the time of ovulation in the breast-feeding mother. Some women begin to ovulate within a month or two of birth; others do not ovulate until six months after they have weaned the baby. And a failure rate of twenty per hundred women per year reflects just that.

Withdrawal.

This means that the man pulls out of the vagina at the last second, just as he feels his orgasm starting, but before ejaculation takes place. Some couples find sexual satisfaction with these gymnastics; most report that the pleasure is less. It fails as a method of birth control because the man's penis leaks out sperm cells even when an ejaculation or orgasm has not occurred—in fact, even when not erect.

Jellies and foams.

Chemical contraceptives are highly effective when compared to nothing or to the methods discussed until now.

They may be used as a cream placed up inside the vagina with a plastic inserter, or as a foam that is similarly inserted into the vagina. These chemical contraceptives are not expensive and are available without a prescription. They should be used a few minutes before intercourse and thus may interfere with the spontaneity of the moment. If an hour goes by, or prior to a second intercourse, another application should be made.

Foams work by providing a surface where the chemicals can immobilize and kill the sperm; they often fail because the cervix is often reached during intercourse and some sperm may be deposited right at the cervical opening.

Condoms.

Having the man wear a sheath over his penis is a good method of contraception. Problems: the man sometimes waits too long to put it on; and even the best condom can break or tear during intercourse. Besides being a relatively good method of birth control, the condom protects against the transmission of venereal disease.

Diaphragm with jelly or cream.

The diaphragm is a tiny, bowl-shaped device made of rubber. Contraceptive jelly or cream is placed in the bowl and it is inserted into the vagina prior to intercourse. This device must be fitted by your doctor, and frequently cannot be fitted properly at your postpartum checkup, but must be fitted after you have had intercourse a few times to make sure that your vagina will not undergo further changes.

The diaphragm is inserted before intercourse starts and must be left in place for six or more hours afterward, so that the cream or jelly will have a chance to immobilize and kill the sperm.

When the diaphragm fails, it is usually because during sexual excitement in the woman the vagina can change its dimensions greatly, allowing the diaphragm to slip about. The diaphragm has a further disadvantage in that it gives you a chore which must be done after each intercourse: you have to wait six or more hours, and then remove your diaphragm, wash it, dry it, powder the rubber so that it won't deteriorate, and then remember where you store it for the next time you use it.

Most women have enough chores in their lives without adding others.

Intrauterine devices.

These are tiny devices that are called IUDs for short. Sometimes they are called loops or coils because of their shapes, but IUD is a more representative term. They are made of plastic or silastic rubber and sometimes have copper parts. They are inserted by your doctor into your uterus through the cervix.

The exact method of action of the IUD is not known, but it is known that ovulation takes place in the usual way, and that sperm swim by them and reach the fallopian tubes. But in some way the sperm lose their ability to fertilize the egg.

The failure rate is two per hundred women per year, and they probably fail because they fail to change the sperm in some instances. This means that they probably fail for a given man, not for a given woman.

The device can be inserted at your postpartum visit with hardly any discomfort, because the uterus, having recently been dilated with a pregnancy, hardly reacts to the tiny device. However, if you are having cramps, which sometimes occur in the postpartum period, your doctor may choose to wait another month or two in order for your uterus to involute more fully. Sometimes women get cramps when IUDs are inserted, or afterward. If this occurs, be sure to tell your doctor so he can give you some medication.

The disadvantage of the IUD is related to its local activity within the uterus. It can cause spotting and increased flow at menstruation. There is no way to predict how a given woman will react ahead of time. Just remember that if you try an IUD you are not making a life-long commitment; you are just trying it, to see how your own body will react to it.

Contraceptive injection.

A long-action, progesterone-type hormone that is given every three months is now available and is excellent for preventing pregnancies. However, it has certain disadvantages that limit its use.

First, it requires an injection every three months, which ties you to the doctor's office more than most people would like.

Second, many women spot continually with this method, while others stop menstruating. This is not harmful, but it may bother you.

Third, it acts by shutting off the cycling action of the hypothalamus, much like birth control pills, and a small percentage of women receiving the injection do not cycle spontaneously again. This means that they do not ovulate spontaneously again and cannot become pregnant without treatment in the future.

Since this injection can interfere with future fertility, it should be used primarily in women who are fairly certain that they do not want any more children, or in women who cannot use any of the less complicated methods of birth control.

Birth control pills.

When taken as directed, the pill is 100 percent effective in preventing pregnancy. It acts by temporarily stopping the ovulation cycle, and also has a direct action on the cervical mucus, making it a barrier to sperm passage. Failures, or pregnancies, are related to women forgetting their pill schedule, and then not using an alternate method of birth control in order to compensate for the pill error.

The disadvantage of pills is that they do act systemically, and not just locally, and thus can cause side effects in many systems. They can cause nausea, breast swelling, spotting between periods, water retention, and they are usually blamed for any symptoms that occur in the person taking the pill. Often having your doctor switch you to another brand will eliminate any side effect.

Other women find taking the pills gets *rid* of life-long symptoms of cramps, heavy menstrual flow, and premenstrual breast engorgement.

Birth control pills seem to cause high blood pressure in a small percentage of women, so when you start on them you should have your physician check your blood pressure periodically to make sure yours has not gone up. In most women there is no effect on blood pressure at all.

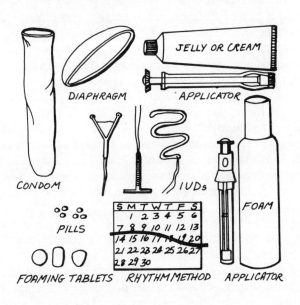

DIAPHRAGM   JELLY OR CREAM   APPLICATOR

CONDOM   IUDs   FOAM

PILLS

FOAMING TABLETS   RHYTHM METHOD   APPLICATOR

Also there seems to be a slightly higher percentage of strokes in women on the pill, but this percentage is *lower* than the number of strokes in women in pregnancy.

There is no way to predict who will get what symptoms with a particular pill. You must realize that with pills, as with IUDs, you are merely trying them when you use them, to see if they agree with you as an individual. They agree well with most people.

Sterilization.

The only other 100-percent-effective method of contraception is sterilization. If you have definitely decided that you do not want any children or that you have as many now as you wish to have, sterilization is logical. The operations have become very popular and are now relatively simple to get. In fact, they are now second only to the pill as the method used by couples desiring no more children, the number of sterilizations having increased more than 200 percent in 1973–1974!

The operations are legal everywhere. If you definitely want one and a doctor does not want to give you one, stand on your rights and insist he refer you to someone who will do the procedure.

In fact, if a hospital denies you the right to a sterilization operation, you can sue them. The Association for Voluntary Sterilization reports that Janet Stein, a twenty-nine-year-old mother of three, was denied the facilities of Northern Westchester Hospital in Mt. Kisco, New York, for a tubal ligation that her obstetrician and she wished to have accomplished at the time of the birth of her third child. The hospital had a rule of prohibiting such procedure on a woman under age thirty in the absence of a threat to her health, unless she already had at least five children. Ms. Stein commenced an action in the United States District Court in the Southern District of New York, and the hospital, shortly thereafter, permitted her doctor to admit her and perform the surgery.

The simplest procedure is a vasectomy done in men. In a ten-minute operation done in the doctor's office under local anesthetic, the tubes that carry the sperm to the penis are cut.

A vasectomy does not remove anything from your sexual organs and does not decrease sexual drive or enjoyment in any way, according to studies we have so far.

A woman can also have a sterilization operation. She can have a hysterectomy (removal of the uterus). Or she can have her tubes tied off or cut. A new, simple method for sealing off the fallopian tubes, which transport the eggs to the uterus, is available in most hospitals. It is called laparoscopic sterilization. It is a safe procedure in which two tiny incisions are made in the abdomen, one for an instrument put in to see through, and the other for an instrument that seals off the tubes.

An estimated one million contraceptive sterilizations are being performed in the U.S. every year now (seven hundred fifty thousand vasectomies and two hundred fifty thousand tubal sterilizations).

Where to get contraceptives or advice.

Your private physician can write a prescription for you to buy pills or insert an IUD or can fit you with the proper size of diaphragm. Some contraceptives such as condoms, creams, and jellies can be bought in a drugstore without a prescription.

Or you may go to a Planned Parenthood clinic. They will counsel patients on various methods, will supply contraceptives, and in some Planned Parenthood clinics will perform sterilization procedures for those who wish them.

Also check with your county health departments or with clinics supported by federal funding to see if you are eligible for their birth control services. These clinics will be listed in the telephone book under United States Department of Health, Education and Welfare. You'll have to check eligibility requirements since some of these will serve only patients below certain income levels.

What about Medicaid coverage?

The Medicaid rules and practices on coverage for family planning services, information, or supplies are confusing. In fact, according to Planned Parenthood officials, in most states less than one out of five women eligible to receive family planning help through Medicaid are actually receiving it. This is despite the law requiring that state welfare agencies offer family planning services to all appropriate public assistance recipients.

What are the oldest methods of birth control?

Coitus interruptus, or withdrawal before emission, is the oldest form of birth control and is mentioned in the book of Genesis. Prescriptions have been found for contraceptive compounds dating back to the Egyptians in 1850 B.C. One calls for a combination of honey and natron, a native sodium carbonate, and another prescribes eating the seeds of a castor-oil plant.

Condoms were used for the prevention of conception as early as the sixteenth century; diaphragms and cervical caps were not in use until the nineteenth century. The rhythm method first received Papal approval in 1930.

I would like to know more about what birth control pills really are.

Oral contraceptives, or birth control pills, are synthetic hormones manufactured in tablet form that act on the hypothalamus in the brain, preventing it from sending out hormones that normally stimulate the ovaries, thus preventing release of the egg from the ovary. Without this ovulation, pregnancy cannot occur.

The pills contain synthetic estrogen or synthetic progestogen hormones, or both. These are the hormones that are secreted in the natural female reproductive cycle. Estrogen is secreted throughout the natural cycle, while progesterone, the natural form of progestogen, is secreted from about day fourteen to about day twenty-six of the menstrual cycle.

What about the side effects from birth control pills?

The side effects most often attributed to birth control tablets are weight gain, nausea, breast tenderness, fluid retention, and the spotting or breakthrough bleeding in the middle of the menstrual cycle. (But sometimes this occurs because you skip a pill or double up.)

Some women on the other hand have these very same problems normally and find they are *corrected* by taking birth control pills.

Often if you have side effects in reaction to one pill, as we noted earlier, you can use a different brand of pill and the problem will disappear.

You will also find that on the pill you may have a shorter and scantier menstrual flow. You will probably have increased cervical discharge, and so need to wash well around the clitoris and vaginal opening whenever you take a shower or bath.

Are there any times you should not take the pill?

A patient who at any time has had thrombophlebitis or who has had problems with the blood clots of thrombosis in pregnancies should not be on the pill.

If at any time you get many severe headaches, or any visual disturbances not noted before being on oral contraceptives, you should immediately get off the pill and see your doctor. Also watch for neurologic signs such as tingling or momentary loss of feeling in a finger. Signs of thrombosis are redness in a leg or pain. In such cases, the woman should be taken off the pill immediately and permanently, and the thrombosis treated.

If you want to go off the pill to become pregnant, what should you do?

You can stop the pill at the end of a pill cycle and try to become pregnant immediately. However, it is wiser to use an alternate method of birth control for that first cycle, such as condoms, and to wait until after the first spontaneous menstrual period in order to become pregnant. This is because the first ovulation after stopping birth control pills is quite variable, occurring at any time from two weeks later to two months later. If you become pregnant with the first ovulation you will have difficulty in defining the starting point of your pregnancy and consequently your due date will be merely an estimate.

It is very helpful to know with accuracy when your baby is due so that your doctor will know if your labor is premature or on time, or if the pregnancy is postmature with the attendant risks and hazards.

Can I get pregnant after the baby if I'm still bleeding?

The first ovulation after giving birth can occur at any time, and in some new mothers occurs while there is still a discharge. It is an old wives' tale that you can't get pregnant while you are bleeding. And many of these old wives were delivering babies more or less every ten months just because they did not use contraceptives while they were still bleeding.

Are there any contraceptives you should not use after having a baby?

All the birth control methods we have discussed are applicable to the postpartum period, with the following slight modifications.

The diaphragm should be fitted after you have had intercourse for about a month, to make sure that the muscles of your vagina have become normally functional.

For the intrauterine device your doctor will want to be sure that your uterus has involuted and is properly firm so that he will not injure the uterus during insertion. The uterus of most breast-feeding mothers will usually be ready by the fourth week after the baby, but some will have to return after one additional month.

Birth control pills can be started immediately unless you are breast-feeding. In this case you must wait until the milk is well established, since early in the postpartum period the estrogen of the birth control pills can inhibit hormones that stimulate lactation. Most nursing mothers can safely start birth control pills by the tenth week. Certainly, if you see the milk supply reduce and you think it's due to the pills, you can stop the pills immediately. Remember that starting any method of birth control is just a trial, not a commitment.

What is a morning-after pill?

The morning-after pill is actually a series of estrogen pills that you take starting the morning after a contraceptive indiscretion, or if you have a sudden change of heart.

This series of high-dose estrogen pills causes the lining of the uterus to change so that a newly fertilized ovum will not have any place to implant properly.

It is not a good method of routine birth control since high doses of estrogen are needed to establish the desired effect in the uterine lining. The doses of estrogen in this pill are so high that most people taking them have severe nausea and even vomiting.

Making the choice.

Decisions concerning what contraceptive to use should be made by you and your husband together. Ask him to read this chapter, then talk over different methods, the failure and success of each in really preventing pregnancy, and how each fits into your life-style.

The following table summarizes the failure rates and times of usage for the different kinds of contraceptives to help you in your choice.

Before you consider the various methods in the table, you should understand what failure rate means. Failure rate for a given method of birth control is the number of pregnancies that occur in one hundred women who use that method over one year's time. If someone leaves out her diaphragm and becomes pregnant, she is excluded from the study. So don't look at that table and say to yourself that those statistics don't apply to you because you will be more responsible. Those statistics do apply to you because they refer to people who are totally responsible for their method of birth control.

METHOD	FAILURE RATE IN PREGNANCIES per 100 women per year	USAGE
Douching	40	each intercourse
Rhythm	25	
Breast-Feeding	20	
Withdrawal	20	each intercourse
Jellies and Foams	10	each intercourse

Condoms	6	each intercourse
Diaphragm and Jelly	5	each intercourse
Intrauterine Device	2	inserted once
Injection	½	every 3 months
Pills	0	taken daily
Sterilization	0	performed once

How to beat the failure rate.

The theories of statistical probabilities may seem far removed from sex in the bedroom, but they can be a valuable method of making more sure that you don't get pregnant.

The trick—to combine birth control methods.

The statistics fit in as a way to tell you just how much better the combination is in preventing pregnancy than a single method of birth control.

Statistical studies show us that if you know the probability of an event happening from one factor, and you know the probability of the event happening from a second factor, you can find the chances of the event happening with both factors by multiplying.

To figure the chances of failure with condoms and a diaphragm together you would multiply as follows: 6/100 times 5/100 = 30/10,000. The chance of pregnancy would then be 0.3 per hundred. So the combination of condom and diaphragm gives you a method which is better than an IUD, but is not as good as pills. The situation isn't completely comparable though, since condom plus diaphragm requires chores for both you and your husband each time you have intercourse, making it less convenient than pills.

But this knowledge of statistics can help you in certain special situations also. If you are breast-feeding and want to wait for a few months before you start pills, you might want to be considering the use of foam until then. Using the chart you see your chance of becoming pregnant will be 20/100 times 10/100 = 200/10,000 or two pregnancies in one hundred women who do this for a year. This calculation should afford you a sense of relief and should enable you to lead a relaxed sexual life until you start your pills.

16

Childbirth Without Bankruptcy—How to Handle Money Matters

Before your baby is even born, he is already running up bills. And the older he gets, day by day, the more the bills start piling up.

You have the obstetrician to pay, the hospital bill for both you and the baby, all those cute baby clothes, the new baby bed and nursery furniture, the diapers, the sterilizer. You wonder whether your bank account will be able to take it.

What does it really cost to get a baby off the ground? And are there things you can do to cut the costs, or at least get as much for your money as possible?

Obstetrician costs.

The bill from your obstetrician can vary widely depending on where you live. If you go to a clinic, the costs will run about the same as going to a private obstetrician.

In both cases, private obstetrician or clinic, the bill covers the prenatal visits, the delivery in the hospital, the care in the hospital, and the checkup six weeks afterward.

Be sure to go in for all of your prenatal and postnatal checkups. They are part of the package you paid for, so you save nothing by skipping these visits, and they are absolutely vital to the health of both you and your baby.

Considering the package of services you get, the bill for the obstetrician is quite a bargain. He is on call twenty-four hours a day for nine months and six weeks in return for his fee. But if you truly are under economic hardship and cannot afford to pay that much, talk it over with your doctor. He may be willing to reduce his fee, or he certainly will be willing to let you pay it in several payments.

Hospital costs.

Hospital costs continue to go up and up, mostly because wages keep going up, and the biggest outlay of capital for hospitals is in wages for personnel. Average cost per hospital day can now reach a hundred and fifty dollars—and still counting. So your hospital bill will include about six hundred dollars for your bed if you stay four days, more if you stay longer, nursery charges, plus charges for the delivery room, for anesthetic if you use it, and for any medications or X rays if you needed them. If you have a telephone or television, there is usually an extra charge for them also.

The grand total is usually around eight hundred dollars, but it can go up or down from that depending on what part of the country you live in, what kind of a hospital you go to, and how long you stay.

The pediatrician.

A pediatrician, whether your own whom you have already selected for your baby or one of the hospital staff, will be performing some services in the hospital. He will give your new baby a checkup to see that he is completely normal and healthy. He'll check him and his charts to see that he is faring well during the first few days in the hospital nursery. The circumcision, if desired, will be performed by the obstetrician at an additional charge.

Later you will be taking your baby in for regular checkups to a pediatrician or a well-baby clinic. The usual schedule is a checkup every month for the first six months, then every six months after that. These checkups are absolutely vital to the health and well-being of your baby so that you know that he is developing properly; and under no circumstances should you try to save money by skipping these appointments. Your baby will have a detailed schedule of immunizations, which the pediatrician will outline.

If you do not have a pediatrician, check with your obstetrician for a recommendation of someone in your area he thinks is particularly good. Or ask him about a well-baby clinic near you. It is important that your pediatrician or clinic be fairly near you and convenient to get to because you will be going there fairly frequently.

Again, fees vary according to what part of the country you live in.

All the other costs.

What else you spend is going to depend a great deal on you and how much you really want to save. Your maternity outfit can consist of a couple of pairs of slacks and skirts, and an assortment of tops, or it can be an elaborate designer wardrobe with a different outfit every day. Your baby's layette can be of the finest fabrics with lace and hand embroidery, or it can consist of the essentials that he or she is really going to use.

The nursery furniture can be the most expensive you can find, or you can make do with a second-hand crib, one chest for storage, and a refinished, sturdy kitchen table for dressing the baby on.

Will health insurance cover medical costs?

If you have health insurance, either privately or at your job or your husband's job, many of your new baby costs will be covered. Check over your policies carefully to make sure what is covered and what is not. Many people don't even claim the moneys coming to them because they don't know what they're entitled to.

Coverage varies tremendously. For example, within Blue Cross there are some seventy-four separate organizations, each setting its own policy. In some plans, Blue Cross insurance will pay the full hospital bill; in others it will pay part; some Blue Cross plans include no maternity benefits at all.

And here's one for you. If you are not married and are a dependent daughter of a person who is insured, in some plans Blue Cross will pay up to seven days in the hospital for delivery of a baby. But even if you are under twenty-one, if you get married you will not be covered under that policy.

If you are married less than nine months, sometimes ten, most policies will not make any maternity payments.

If you are working at a company with an insurance plan that does not cover maternity care, unless there are other career advantages to where you are working, it can pay if you are planning to have a baby to change to another job where maternity benefits are covered.

If your income is low enough, you may be able to qualify for Medicaid. In most states, Medicaid will pay the entire delivery cost for those eligible.

States vary on their requirements. In some states, you can earn as much as $3,500 a year and have money in the bank and still be eligible for it. In other states you have to be on public assistance. Call your local Medicaid office if you think you might be eligible. In fact, you might call twice since sometimes Medicaid employees aren't too sure about all the eligibility clauses themselves.

Health insurance tips.

You can pick up maternity benefits after your pregnancy has started by transferring from a nonfamily to a family group plan at most jobs.

If you and your husband have separate policies it is ethical and moral to apply to both for benefits. After all, you both paid premiums.

Advice on buying health insurance.

If you don't have health insurance and are planning on having a child, or even already have a family, you will want to look over various plans carefully to make sure that your coverage is best for your needs. Group insurance policies are cheaper if you are eligible for them.

The American Academy of Pediatrics, an organization representing more than twelve thousand pediatricians in the U.S., has developed the following guidelines to help you select a good family health insurance program. Whether you are buying a health insurance policy privately and want to get the best protection at the least cost, or whether you want to check out the adequacy of your policy at work, look over these guidelines.

FEATURES ESSENTIAL TO ANY SOUND HEALTH INSURANCE PROGRAM

1. All family members should be covered equally, including each child, from birth.

2. All major medical and surgical expenses should be covered.

3. Protection from catastrophic health expenses should be covered.

4. When the subscriber terminates his employment, he should be able to convert and continue his health insurance policy.

5. Exclusions (what is *not* covered) should be clearly identified and easy to understand.

6. If coinsurance, corridors, or deductibles are part of the policy, you may have costs in addition to your premium. Ask your agent to explain such provisions.

PRIORITIES

The following benefits should be provided in a comprehensive medical insurance policy.

FIRST PRIORITIES

1. Medical care, including health supervision and preventive care performed and supervised by a physician in or out of the hospital.

2. Surgical care performed in or out of the hospital, plastic or reconstructive surgery where medically indicated.

3. Pregnancy and all complications, including care of the unborn child.

4. Care of the newborn infant, including the premature, *from birth.* (Many policies exclude infants from coverage for fourteen to thirty days after birth.)

5. Laboratory and pathological services requested by a physician and performed in an approved laboratory.

6. X-ray services in or out of the hospital.

7. Radiation therapy in or out of the hospital.

8. Anesthesia services in or out of the hospital.

9. Consultations in or out of the hospital.

10. Services rendered by more than one physician for the same illness or during the same hospitalization.

11. Inhalation and physical therapy under the direction of a physician.

12. Medication expenses while in a hospital, and other medication expenses beyond an annual deductible out of the hospital.

13. Emergency psychiatric care.

14. Emergency ambulance service.

15. Extended care services ordered by a physician.

16. Prosthetic appliances; braces.

SECOND PRIORITIES

1. Psychiatric services.
2. Podiatry.
3. Rental and purchases of medical equipment.
4. Psychological testing.

THIRD PRIORITIES

1. Cosmetic surgery (elective).
2. Organ transplants.
3. Eyeglasses.

4. Social services, if beneficial.

Dental care is important to your child's health; you may want to investigate the possibility of obtaining coverage for such care.

REDUCING THE COST OF HEALTH INSURANCE

The type of policy containing most of these recommendations is termed comprehensive major medical insurance. Such policies almost always include a deductible, which is the part of your medical costs you must pay before the insurance starts to pay. As in automobile insurance, the larger the deductible, the smaller your insurance premium will be. The deductible should apply to a family's total yearly medical expenses; if the deductible is linked to each illness or to each family member, the amount you may have to pay in addition to your premium becomes unpredictable. Health supervision and preventive medicine are essential to good medical care and should be included in the insurance coverage as part of a deductible.

A model newborn insurance bill.

A model law requiring health insurance coverage for newborn infants from the moment of birth has also been developed by the American Academy of Pediatrics.

The model bill, developed with the assistance of the Health Insurance Association of America, is designed to help groups of pediatricians and others to get new insurance laws. In dozens of states now, insurance coverage usually excludes the newborn for periods ranging from the first fourteen to the first ninety days.

The model law provides that all types of health insurance policies covering dependents include coverage for the newborn infant from the moment of birth. The coverage would include treatment for injury, sickness, congenital defects, and birth abnormalities.

In the forty-three states that do not have such a law, a substantial proportion of policies issued do not provide such coverage.

"We don't think that young couples should be penalized

for having a child with a major problem," Donald Schiff, M.D., chairman of the pediatrician's committee forming the plan, says. "We're looking for a way to help parents pay for this expensive kind of care."

Academy chapters have been active in promoting passage of newborn insurance legislation in the seven states that currently have such laws. Chapters in twenty-six other states are currently working to enact such legislation in their areas.

Costs in Canada.

If you are planning to move to Canada, do it before you have your baby. It's cheaper there. In Nova Scotia, baby delivery costs about thirty dollars less if you go to a general practitioner instead of an obstetrician. In British Columbia hospital beds cost one dollar a day.

Before you move to Canada, arrange for Landed Immigrant Status, showing you are a resident. In Nova Scotia medical care is paid for out of sales taxes. You register with the Maritime Health Services for Medical Services Insurance and with the Nova Scotia Hospital Insurance Commission. This medical insurance will pay for 85 percent of the doctor bills. The hospital room is free if you stay in a ward, as are the medications and the delivery room. If you stay in a private room and have insurance, the room costs you three dollars a day.

In British Columbia on the Pacific Coast, the rules are a bit different. You have to pay premiums on insurance to receive benefits, usually about twelve dollars and fifty cents a month for a family of three.

A child born in Canada of American parents can retain American citizenship or be eligible for Canadian citizenship.

Ways to save on life insurance.

Now that your family has expanded, you will probably be approached by life insurance agents who will urge you to expand your life insurance.

As you consider whether your insurance is adequate or needs redesigning, look over the possible policies carefully and compare their features. There are a number of ways to save costs on your coverage, and insurance agents may not call all of them to your attention.

Here is a list of many money-saving possibilities that may apply to you.

- Semiannual, quarterly, and monthly premiums often cost more than annual premiums. The extra payments on a monthly payment plan may amount to 15 percent more than the annual rate, and the IRS does not consider it interest, so there is no tax deduction for it.

- The person who needs straight life insurance will save money by buying it in a package deal that includes term insurance, which has a cash-in value at the end of a certain time.

- Participating policies (providing dividends) are available from stock companies and mutual companies. They cost a little more at first, but the dividends start adding up, so that after about ten years the overall cost of participating policies tends to be less.

- In New York, Connecticut, or Massachusetts, up to thirty thousand dollars of life insurance can be purchased from savings banks, which have no agents and charge smaller premiums.

- Persons with more straight life coverage than they need can convert some or all of it to a smaller face value of paid-up insurance or "extended term insurance" that may run a number of years—without paying a cent more in premiums.

Ways to save money before and after childbirth.

Despite the high costs of birthing in this country, there are ways to save money and still maintain quality care for yourself and your child. Here are a number of ways we have run into. Read them over. You can probably add a few of your own.

If you are working, keep your job as long as you feel up to it before delivery. Most women feel marvelous during this period, except for being somewhat clumsy and awkward, and there is no reason you shouldn't work right up to the day before you deliver if you feel like it. The Supreme Court recently ruled that schools cannot force teachers who are pregnant to take maternity leave until the last few weeks.

Stop using the medicines in your medicine chest. Any drug or medicine you take has the potential for harming the infant developing in your uterus. Don't take chances. Don't take pills. Vitamins are the only things you should be taking during pregnancy, except for something your doctor specifically recommends. And if you're breast-feeding your baby, you shouldn't be taking anything without your doctor's permission either.

Ask your relatives to check their attics. Nostalgia items are very much in vogue now. Besides being great conversation pieces, an old lacy baby outfit or an antique bassinet used by you or your husband when you were babies can have great sentimental value—as well as money-saving value.

Don't stay in the hospital any longer than you have to. You can go home and spend the day in bed and let your husband or a relative or hired help wait on you much more cheaply than staying in bed at the hospital and letting the hospital staff wait on you. Usually the saving of one day in the hospital will pay for a maid for one week at home.

You can usually save 30 percent of your hospital cost in semiprivate accommodations. This can also give you a chance to meet someone with similar immediate concerns and feelings.

Breast-feed your baby. It's easier, more convenient, and less expensive.

Prepare some of your own baby foods instead of buying already prepared ones. What's so hard about squishing up a ripe banana, an avocado, or scraping an apple? It will also save your baby from getting too much salt since baby food manufacturers put an unnecessary amount of salt in baby food that could well be a strain on immature kidneys and a cause of high blood pressure. A blender will puree any vegetable you are having for your meal.

Keep your maternity outfits simple. Most people wear tailored, simple clothes now anyway, so there is no need for an elaborate maternity wardrobe. A few good, basic items will take you anywhere. Don't try to save when it comes to shoes, maternity girdles, or maternity bras, though. These are essential to your comfort and health and are no place to try to save a dollar.

Trade maternity clothes with friends who are also having babies. Or buy them second hand.

Buy your vitamins in large amounts and buy them at discount stores.

Check your local thrift shops. Second-hand stores can have great buys on cribs, sterilizers, chests, and other baby equipment.

Watch the ads in your local newspaper. Not only baby equipment, but baby clothes can be fantastic bargains at house and garage sales. They not only save you money but are fun and a great way to get to know your neighbors.

Refinish old things. An old kitchen table painted or stained for a fresh look, an old chest freshened up with nursery decals, storage shelves made from apple crates painted in bright colors or covered with striped contact paper can make great additions to any new baby's nursery. If you have older children in the family, let them help paint and fix so that they feel part of the new adventure. When you paint, be sure you are not using paint with lead in it. A few flakes a week are enough to kill a baby or make him mentally retarded for life.

Don't buy things for the baby too early. Why buy a sweater now, and get three more for baby presents?

Study decorating and baby magazines. There are many inexpensive ways to decorate a nursery that cost almost nothing. The less furniture, the better. Rely on bright colors.

If you don't want to spend money for a fancy bathtub, simply get an inexpensive plastic babytub (sold in all department stores) and use it to bathe your baby at the kitchen counter or on a table or vanity in the bathroom. (Never bathe him right in the sink. It's too easy for him to hit his head on the faucets, or for the hot water to get turned on accidentally.)

Skip the bassinet. He's only going to use it for a few weeks anyway. Get a regular-sized crib right in the beginning. Use padded side protectors on three sides, and put the fourth one across the crib in the middle to divide it in half and make it cozy. Put baby at the head half of the bed with the pads to protect him from the wood sides of the crib. Use the foot half of the crib (away from him) to store a few extra diapers and changes of everyday clothes.

One of the best ways to save money is to practice preventive medicine. It's always easier—and less costly—to prevent illness or to treat it in the early stages than it is later on when some trouble has become serious.

This is not only good advice for saving money, but also for being the best of new parents. See that you follow your doctor's orders on what he says to do for your baby. Make sure, for example, that the baby goes in for his regular checkups and gets the proper immunization shots. And see that you follow your doctor's orders for what you should do to take care of yourself as a new mother. The best parent in the world is the one who has taken care of herself so that she is well enough, relaxed enough, and happy enough to give her baby love.

Glossary

Here is a glossary of commonly used obstetric, gynecologic, and other medical terms that we think you will find useful.

abortion   Birth of a fetus or embryo before it is able to survive. An abortion may be spontaneous (without chemical or surgical interference) or induced (brought on by surgery or other means).

afterbirth   See **placenta.**

amnion   A thin, transparent sac enclosing the unborn baby and the protective fluid surrounding it.

analgesic   A drug that lessens pain.

androgen   A hormone that produces masculine characteristics or is similar to male hormone.

anesthetic   A drug given by inhalation, by mouth, or by injection that causes loss of pain in a specific area or loss of consciousness.

anovulation   Suspension or cessation of the release of an ovum.

a–z test   Laboratory test of patient's urine to determine pregnancy; named after the two German physicians who developed the test, Selmar Aschheim and Bernhardt Zondek. This test required laboratory animals and it is now obsolete.

b.b.t. (basal body temperature) Temperature of the body at its lowest, usually taken immediately on waking. A rise in b.b.t. is one method used to determine time of ovulation.

birth canal See **vagina**.

blastocyst The early, multicelled form that occurs in the first few days after fertilization.

breech birth Birth of a baby with the buttocks or feet first.

cervical cap A mechanical means of contraception. Closely fitted directly over the cervix, it forms a barrier that prevents sperm from entering the uterus.

cervix The mouth of the uterus, which is that portion of the uterus that projects into the vagina. Its central canal connects the vagina with the uterine cavity.

cesarean section Birth of a baby through surgical incisions made in the mother's abdomen and uterus.

chloasma Discoloration of skin pigment of the face, the so-called "mask of pregnancy." It can also occur in users of birth control pills.

chorionic gonadotropin A hormonal substance produced by the placenta and having effect on the ovary.

circumcision A quick operation to remove a male infant's foreskin.

coitus interruptus Birth control by withdrawal before ejaculation.

conception The union of a sperm from the male and an egg in the female that results in pregnancy; also called fertilization.

condom A sheath covering the penis that is used for contraceptive purposes or to prevent transmission of disease.

contraceptive foam, jellies, and creams Spermicidal products that immobilize or kill sperm by chemical action.

contractions Uterine muscular activity that can occur at any time, whether during pregnancy or not. In pregnancy they occur with increasing frequency as the due date is approached. When there is no pregnancy they are felt as the cramps some women experience during menstruation, or that sometimes occur during sexual activity.

cystitis Inflammation of the bladder.

delivery Act of giving birth.

diaphragm A device of molded rubber that is fitted over the cervix to hold a spermicidal jelly or cream against the cervix.

diuresis Passage of large amounts of urine due to mobilization of fluids from the body.

douche To flush the vagina with water or medicated solution.

due date The approximate expected date of the baby's birth, normally about two hundred eighty days (or about nine months and seven days) from the first day of the last menstrual period. Most people deliver their baby within two weeks on either side of this date.

dysfunction Disturbance, impairment, or abnormality of the behavior of an organ.

eclampsia See **toxemia**.

ectopic pregnancy Growth of the fertilized egg anywhere outside its normal place in the uterus. When the growth occurs in one of the fallopian tubes, it is called a tubal pregnancy.

edema Excessive fluid retention in the body.

embryo The unborn baby during the first three months of gestation; after three months it is called a fetus.

endocrine glands Organs that secrete hormones into the body.

endogenous Developing or originating within your body.

endometriosis A condition in which endometrial tissue develops outside of the uterus, either on the ovaries or elsewhere outside of the uterine cavity. This tissue responds to cyclic hormonal secretions, causing varying degrees of pain or swelling.

endometrium The lining of the uterus. It undergoes continual changes during the monthly cycle.

episiotomy A surgical incision of the tissue between the vagina and the anus to allow more room for the emerging child, thereby preventing excessive stretching and possible tearing of the mother's tissues.

ergonovine A tablet or injection that causes the uterus to contract.

estrogen A hormone secreted by the ovaries that is largely responsible for feminine body characteristics and for changes in the uterus associated with menstruation and pregnancy.

etiology The cause and origin of any disease or process.

exogenous Developing or originating outside your body.

fallopian tubes Two ducts, each one to three inches long, that transport eggs from the ovaries to the uterus. Fertilization takes place here.

false labor Uterine contractions that resemble true labor but are not accompanied by dilation of the cervix or progressive changes leading to birth.

false pregnancy A condition, usually caused by psychological factors, in which a nonpregnant woman experiences the symptoms of pregnancy, including absence of menstruation, breast sensations, nausea, and even swelling of the abdomen.

fertility The capacity to produce offspring; the term is applied to both males and females.

fertilization The union of the sperm and egg to produce a special cell that can develop into embryo and placenta.

fetus An unborn baby after the third month of gestation; prior to the third month it is called an embryo. (This is an arbitrary classification.)

flatus Intestinal gas passed out through the rectum.

follicle stimulating hormone (FSH) A hormone produced by the anterior lobe of the pituitary that acts upon ovaries.

forceps An instrument sometimes used in delivery to grasp the baby's head so that it can be assisted through the birth canal.

genital An organ involved in generation or reproduction. The term also describes the region of reproductive organs.

gonad The sex glands. In the male the testes are the gonads; in the female the ovaries are the gonads.

gonadotropins Gonad-stimulating hormones. In women two of the gonadotropins are FSH and LH.

habitual aborter A woman who has lost three or more successive pregnancies.

histological Pertaining to the microscopic structure of the tissues of organisms.

hormones Secretions of the endocrine glands.

hypermenorrhea Excessive menstrual flow.

hyperplasia Growth of cells in which the growth is excessive or piles up.

hypomenorrhea A reduced amount of menstrual discharge.

implantation The process after fertilization in which the blastocyst burrows into the developed endometrial lining of the uterus.

(This usually occurs sometime in the interval of days eighteen and a half to twenty-three and a half of the menstrual cycle.)

induced labor Labor started through the use of chemical or mechanical aids.

infertility Inability to have offspring.

involute To return to the normal nonpregnant state.

IUCD or IUD (intrauterine contraceptive device) A small object which, when inserted in the uterus, prevents fertilization.

labor The process during which the unborn baby begins to emerge from the uterus and descend into the birth canal.

labor pains Special uterine contractions that occur in a progressive way with increasing strength and frequency, and cause the cervix to dilate. They are better called labor contractions since they do not always hurt.

lanugo Fine, downlike hairs on the skin of a newborn.

libido Sexual desire.

ligament Tough, fibrous band that connects bones or supports organs.

luteinizing hormone (LH) This hormone is produced by the anterior lobe of the pituitary gland in the process of causing ovulation.

mammography X-ray technique for detecting breast cancer or defining breast lumps.

menarche The time in a young woman's life when menstruation begins.

menopause The time in a woman's life when menstruation ceases to occur.

menses The discharge during menstruation, consisting of sloughed-off endometrium plus blood.

menstrual period The bleeding time occurring monthly during which the menses flow.

miscarriage A popular term for spontaneous abortion.

mittelschmerz Pain in the middle of the menstrual cycle, caused by ovulatory changes in the ovary.

monilial vaginitis A vaginal infection caused by a fungus called monilia or candida albicans; itching and discharge are the usual symptoms.

morning sickness Nausea or vomiting that may occur during the first three months of pregnancy.

Moro reflex   A reflex in response to sudden noise or movement in which the newborn convulsively moves its arms and legs.

multipara   A woman who has given birth and is pregnant again.

multiple birth   Two or more children delivered at the same time by one mother.

natal   Referring to birth.

neonatal   Pertaining to the first four weeks of life.

obstetrics   The branch of medicine dealing with pregnancy and childbirth.

oligomenorrhea   Menstruation that is abnormally infrequent or scanty.

os   A mouth or orifice, or the opening into one.

ovary   A gland that produces unfertilized eggs and hormones. There are two ovaries in the female body.

ovulation   The time occurring approximately every twenty-eight days during which an ovum is released from one of the ovaries.

ovum (pl., ova)   The egg cell produced by the ovary.

Papanicolaou test   A method of finding whether malignancy exists by staining a sample of cells from an organ.

pathologic   An abnormal state or condition.

pelvic organs   Organs located within the pelvic cavity. In women these are the uterus, tubes, and ovaries; the lower portions of the intestines; and the urinary bladder.

perinatal   Around the time of birth.

perineum   In the female, the tissue between the vagina and the anus.

phlebitis   A condition in which a vein is inflamed and a thrombus or clot of blood may form at the site of inflammation.

physiologic   Normal, not pathologic.

pituitary gland   An endocrine gland located at the base of the brain consisting of two lobes. The anterior lobe produces hormones that act on the ovaries.

placenta   An oval, spongy structure that forms on the inside wall of the uterus during pregnancy. It passes oxygen and nourishment from the mother to the fetus and waste products from the fetus to the mother via the umbilical cord. Also known as the afterbirth because it is expelled from the uterus soon after delivery.

postnatal   After birth.

postpartum   After delivery.

premature A baby born any time from the twenty-eighth to the thirty-sixth week of pregnancy or weighing five and a half pounds or less at birth.

premenstrual tension A complex of physical and psychological symptoms preceding the menses.

prenatal Before birth.

prepared childbirth Childbirth using special techniques of breathing and relaxation during labor and delivery that reduce or eliminate the need for analgesics or anesthetics.

prepartal Before delivery.

primary amenorrhea Failure of menstruation to occur at puberty.

primipara A woman who has given birth once.

progesterone The hormone that prepares the uterus for reception and development of a fertilized egg.

prolactin A hormone secreted by the anterior pituitary that stimulates lactation or milk production.

proliferate To grow by reproduction of similar cells.

proliferative phase The phase of the endometrial lining that starts with the onset of menstruation and is stimulated by estrogen. During this time, until about "day fourteen," the endometrium thickens, glands form, and the supply of blood vessels increases.

psychogenic Having an emotional or psychological origin as opposed to an organic basis.

quickening The first noticeable movements of the unborn baby, usually during the fourth or fifth month. If you add twenty-two weeks to your quickening date you get a good estimate of when you are due.

rabbit test See **a–z test.**

regression A returning to an earlier state.

reproductive cycle The interval between one menses and the next, lasting an average of twenty-eight days.

Rh factor A property of blood cells found in 85 percent of human beings. Individuals who have the Rh factor are called Rh-positive; those without the factor are termed Rh-negative.

rhythm method Birth control by temporary abstinence at a time when ovulation is most likely to occur.

rooming-in Hospital program that allows the baby to share the mother's room.

secondary amenorrhea Cessation of menstruation after it has once been established at puberty.

secretory phase The phase of the endometrial lining that occurs after ovulation under the influence of progesterone, the hormone produced with ovulation. In this phase the endometrial glands begin to secrete nourishing substances in preparation for implantation.

sperm (spermatozoa) The sperm cells.

sterility Inability to conceive. This may be temporary or permanent.

steroid An organic chemical that is fat-soluble. Sex hormones, among other compounds, are steroids.

stillborn Born dead.

syndrome A series of symptoms and findings that together make up a disease picture.

tampon An absorbent, small pad worn inside the vagina to absorb menstrual flow.

testosterone Male sex hormone.

toxemia An illness of late pregnancy characterized by rapid weight gain, increasing blood pressure, severe headaches, and occasionally eclampsia (convulsions and coma). Eclampsia usually can be prevented by proper prenatal care.

trichomoniasis A vaginal infection, producing a discharge, that is caused by the organism trichomonas vaginalis.

trimester A three-month time period; the nine months of pregnancy are divided into the first, second, and third trimesters.

tubal pregnancy See **ectopic pregnancy.**

umbilical cord A tubelike structure that carries oxygen and nourishment from the placenta to the fetus and waste products from the fetus to the placenta; the cord is severed by the attendant at birth, and its stump forms the baby's navel.

umbilicus The naval (belly button).

uterine cavity Space within the uterus.

uterus (womb) The organ that carries the developing fetus.

vagina The canal between the uterus and the exterior of the female body.

vernix White, cheeselike material that covers and protects the baby's skin in the uterus.

vulva The external female genital organs.

witches' milk   Small quantities of milk that may be secreted from the newborn's nipples due to the effects of the mother's natural pregnancy hormones.

zygote   The fertilized egg.

Index

About the Authors

DR. GIDEON G. PANTER is an obstetrician and gynecologist in private practice in New York City. He graduated from Cornell University College of Medicine and served his residency at Columbia-Presbyterian Medical Center in New York. He is now assistant clinical professor of obstetrics and gynecology at the New York Hospital–Cornell Medical Center, is a diplomate of the American Board of Obstetrics and Gynecology, and has served on the board of directors of the American Society for Psychoprophylaxis in Obstetrics.

SHIRLEY MOTTER LINDE is a well-known author with a dozen books and hundreds of magazine and newspaper features among her credits. Her most recent books include *Sickle Cell: A Complete Guide; The Complete Allergy Guide; Orthotherapy; You Don't Have To Ache; High Blood Pressure: What Causes It, How to Tell If You Have It, How to Control It for a Longer Life;* and *The Sleep Book: Current Research, Dream Interpretations, Folk Lore, Fantasy, Myth, Facts and Questions Relating to the Subject of Sleep.*.